ITALIAN
Cookbook 2022

300 EASY & TASTY EVERYDAY RECIPES FOR YOU AND YOUR FAMILY

Maria Lacuoca

© Copyright 2022 by Maria Lacuoca - All rights reserved.

The content contained within this book may not be reproduced, duplicated or transmitted without direct written permission from the author or the publisher.

Under no circumstances will any blame or legal responsibility be held against the publisher, or author, for any damages, reparation, or monetary loss due to the information contained within this book. Either directly or indirectly.

Legal Notice:

This book is copyright protected. This book is only for personal use. You cannot amend, distribute, sell, use, quote or paraphrase any part, or the content within this book, without the consent of the author or publisher.

Disclaimer Notice:

Please note the information contained within this document is for educational and entertainment purposes only. All effort has been executed to present accurate, up to date, and reliable, complete information. No warranties of any kind are declared or implied. Readers acknowledge that the author is not engaging in the rendering of legal, financial, medical or professional advice. The content within this book has been derived from various sources. Please consult a licensed professional before attempting any techniques outlined in this book.

By reading this document, the reader agrees that under no circumstances is the author responsible for any losses, direct or indirect, which are incurred as a result of the use of information contained within this document, including, but not limited to, errors, omissions, or inaccuracies.

Table of Contents

Chapter 1. Italian Cooking: Overview and History 7

Chapter 2. The Main Ingredients in Italian Cooking 11

Breakfast 13
- Italian Breakfast Casseroles 13
- Italian Mini Frittatas 13
- Egg And Tomato Scramble 14
- Breakfast Pizza Skillet 14
- Breakfast Risotto 15
- Italian Strata 15
- Meatball Sandwich....................16
- Calico Pepper Frittata............16
- Egg And Tomato Scramble 17
- Breakfast Couscous 17
- Caramelized Mushroom And Onion Frittata........................18
- Cheesy Vegetable Frittata 18
- Creamy Breakfast Oatmeal.. 18
- Chicken 'n' Ham Frittata 19
- Ricotta Pancakes 19
- Italian Brunch Torte 20
- Simple Italian Omelete 20

Pasta..22
- Penne Pasta with Spinach and Bacon................................22
- Pasta with Lentils....................22
- White Lasagna with mushrooms........................23
- Spaghetti Picchi Pacchiu 23
- Baked Ziti 24
- Spaghetti With Clams 24
- Artichoke Spinach Lasagna... 25
- Pasta with Zucchini and Shrimp 25
- Vegetarian Cabbage Rolls ... 26
- Vermicelli With Tomato Sauce.....26
- Classic Baked Pasta 27
- Milanese Risotto 28
- Pasta Fagioli.............................28
- Spaghetti with Garlic Sauce.. 28
- Spaghetti with Clam Sauce ... 29
- Spaghetti with Tomato Sauce 29
- Veal Cutlets with Tomato and Basil Sauce......................29
- Sicilian Eggplant Rigatoni 30
- Pasta with Cannellini Beans . 30
- Maccheroni with Cauliflower 31
- Lentil Bolognese........................31
- Pasta with Garlic and Oil 32
- Green Tomato Pasta 32
- Pasta with Bread Crumbs...... 32
- Pistachio Pasta........................33
- Norcina Style Pasta................. 33
- Eggplant Pasta 34
- Baked Stuffed Shells................ 34
- Tofu Spinach Lasagna 35
- Italian Lasagna 35
- Italian Savory Bread Pasta 36
- Italian Shrimp Caprese Pasta 36
- Fusilli with Chicken RAGÙ 37
- Pepperoni Pasta 37
- Baked Elbows with Pork RAGÙ...38
- No-bake Mushroom Lasagna 38
- Braised Octopus with Spaghetti 39
- Spinach Tortelloni..................... 40
- Special Italian Easter Pizza ... 41

Rice..42
- Classic Paella Simple 42
- Rice Balls 43
- Lemon-Rice Soup 43
- Rice with Olives........................ 44
- Basil Rice 44
- Rice Cake................................... 45
- Cold Rice in Aspic 45
- Hot Rice Salad 46
- Italian Rice Pie........................ 46
- Italian Rice with Porcini mushrooms 46
- Milanese-Style Risotto 47
- Italian Rice with Saffron & Parmesan 47
- Rice with Potatoes and Leeks 48
- Creamy Rice with Porcini 48
- Italian Jasmine Rice 48

Soups..49
- Lentil Soup................................. 49
- Garden Minestrone Soup 49
- Italian Beef Stew...................... 50
- Basil Spaghetti Soup 50
- Chickpea Soup 51
- Recipe Italian Wedding Soup 51
- Escarole and Bean Soup......... 52
- Sausage, Potato and Kale Soup... 52
- Cream Of Tomato Soup 52
- Garlic Tomato Soup 53
- Slow Cooked Vegetable Soup 53
- Braised Oxtail Stew 54
- Quick Italian Vegetable Soup 54
- Zucchini Tomato Soup............. 55
- Fish stock 55
- Mixed Meat Stock.................... 56
- Broccoli Soup............................. 56
- Cauliflower and Tomato Soup 57
- Tuscan Bean Soup..................... 57
- Italian Potato Soup................... 58
- Rice and Potato Soup 58
- Roman "Egg Drop" Soup......... 59
- Bell Pasta Soup 59
- Beef Soup................................. 59
- Smokey Mediter- Soup 60
- Italian Halibut Chowder.......... 60

Bread and Pizza..........................62
- Pizza Dough 62
- Italian Herbed Pizza Dough.. 62
- Shaved Asparagus, Ricotta, and Oven-roasted Tomato Pizza........ 63
- Beef Soup................................. 63
- Italian Easter Bread 64
- Basil Tomato Bread 64
- Dilly Onion Bread 65
- Roasted Garlic Bread 65
- Sausage, Potato and Kale Soup... 65
- Italian Herb Bread 66

Artichoke Pizza........................... 66
Trenton Tomato Pie Pizza...... 67
Italian Garlic Bread 67
Carrot Pizza With Fontina And Red Onion................................. 68
Herb Bread 68
Eggplant, Tomato, And Fontina Pizza.. 69
Quick Italian Vegetable Soup 70
Basic Focaccia with Basil 70
Ciabatta Bread......................... 71
Roman "Egg Drop" Soup......... 71
Crusty Hoagie Bread................ 72
Bell Pasta Soup 72
Smokey Mediter- Soup 73
Italian Halibut Chowder........... 73

Vegetables.....................................74
Zucchini Pesto......................... 74
Horseradish Mashed Potatoes Side Dish 74
Zesty Zucchini 74
Green Bean in Bread Crumbs 75
Italian Garlic Mushrooms 75
Balsamic Roasted Vegetables 75
Vegetarian Strata 76
Eggplant Parmesan 76
Broccoli Flan with Anchovy Sauce 77
Spinach Manicotti with Italian Sausage..................................... 77
Turnip Greens and Pancetta. 78
Zucchini Crepes 78
Italian-Style Baked Zucchini 79
Whole Braised Cauliflower... 79
Zucchini With Anchovies And Capers 80
Pan Fried Asparagus 80
Easy Baked Mushrooms 80
Stuffed Cabbage....................... 81
Cool Cucumber Pasta 81
Roast Tuscan Potatoes 82
Stuffed Mushroom 82
Italian Stewed Tomatoes 82
Tomato Onion Quiche............. 83
Crispy Cauliflower.................... 83

Fried Peppers with Potatoes 84
Asparagus With Fresh Basil Sauce 84
Italian Style Green Beans 84
Stewed Eggplant and Tomatoes.. 85
Eggplant Bruschetta................ 85
Italian Peas 85
Italian Kale 86
Eggplant Cutlets 86
Gnocchi 86

Fish and Seafood 87
Venice Fish Fillets 87
Fettuccini and Salmon 87
Peppered Mussels 87
Herb-Grilled Salmon 88
Lobster Tail with Tomato Confit and Basil Oil.............................. 88
Filet of Sole Francese 89
Italian Christmas Eel............... 89
Combined Fried Fish 90
Cioppino 90
Deviled Shrimp 90
Creamy Presto Shrimp 91
Monkfish in Leek Sauce with Italian Olives 91
Bluefish Alla Lucia 91
Almond and Pistachio-crusted Brownish-yellow Jack Steak with Artichoke Salad 92
Garlic-and-herb-braised Squid.... 92
Cod with Potatoes................... 93
Swordfish in Red Sauce 93
White Bean Crostini 93
Mediterranean Style Salmon 94
Spicy Shrimp & Peppers With Pasta 94
Baked Clams Oreganata 95
Piccata Cod 95

Meat (Poultry, Beef, Pork and Lamb)..96
Lemon Chicken 96
Zucchini and Corn-stuffed Chicken 96
Sausage, Peppers, Onion, And Potato Bake 97

Braised Lamb Shanks 97
Roast Sicilian Rabbit................ 98
Easy Beef Braciole................... 98
Cube Steak Parmesan............. 99
Roasted Calabrian Chicken .. 99
Chicken Fettuccini Alfredo . 100
Roast Chicken With Rosemary..... 100
Italian Lamb 101
Italian Stuffed Chicken Breast..... 101
Lemon Chicken Piccata 102
Beef Braised in Barolo Wine 102
Balsamic Vinegar Steak........ 103
Chicken Milano 103
Parmesan Chicken Bake....... 103
Garlic Tomato Sauce and Meatballs 104
Buffalo Mozzarella and Semi-Candied Tomatoes.................. 105
Pork with Olives 105
Pan Chicken with Tomato.... 105
Italian Frittata ham 106
Turkey Cutlets........................ 106
Lamb Stew With Mint And Apricots... 107
Tunisian-Style Ribs................ 107
Great Meatloaf 108
Italian Pork Tenderloin 108
Simple Braised Beef 109
Spicy Sausage Linguine........ 109
Italian Barbeque Pork Chops..... 110
Beefy Italian Ramen Skillet.110
Quail Stuffed with Mushrooms and Sausage 111
Milan-Style Porkchops 111
Spinach-stuffed Chicken Parmesan 112
Rabbit Stew............................ 112

Eggs and Sauce....................... 113
Marinara Sauce...................... 113
Slim Italian Deviled Eggs 113
Pasta Sauce with Italian Sausage 113
Tuna Sauce............................. 114

Italian Omelet 114
Tomato Sauce 114
Tiramisu...................................115
Spinach Pasta Sauce 115
Italian Cloud Eggs...................115
Mushroom Sausage Omelets 116
Oven-Baked Eggs and Asparagus 116
Crockpot Pasta Sauce With Meat..116
Arrabbiata Sauce 117
Old Italian Meat Sauce 117
Puttanesca Sauce 118
Fettuccine Sauce 118
Pesto Sauce 119
Crockpot Pasta Sauce With Meat..119
Italian Basil Baked Eggs 120
Pizza Sauce..............................120
Italian Egg Toast 120
Scented Deviled Eggs 121
Italian Meat Sauce..................121
Tomato and Basil Sauce 122
Italian Pesto Hollandaise ...122
Clam Sauce 122
Italian Red Sauce....................123
Baked Eggs & Sausage 123
Mexican-Italian Salsa 123
Italian Spaghetti Sauce with Meatballs..................................124
Italian Egg Bake 124
Porcini Mushrooms Sauce ..125
Classic Bolognese Sauce......126

Snacks and Appetizers...............127
Baked Pumpkin Flowers with Ricotta 127
Amaretto Biscotti....................127
Canapes with avocado cream 128
Lentil meatballs 128
Italian Grilled Cheese Sandwich 129
Tomato Fritters 129
Italian Cookies 129
Pizza Biscuits 130

Mussels In Spicy Tomato Sauce 130
Lentil Crostini 131
Roasted Eggplant Spread with Crackers 131
Lettuce and Bread Quiches 132
Swordfish-Stuffed Peppers 132
Pinwheel Pizza Snacks 133
Lobster Salad with Fresh Potatoes 133
Panzanella................................134
Garlic Risotto Stuffed Mushrooms..134

Salads...136
Basil Garden Salad 136
Cherry Tomato Corn Salad .136
Cherry Tomato Salad 137
Arugula Salad With Shaved Parmesan 137
Vegetable Salad 138
Artichoke Red Pepper Tossed Salad 138
Copper Carrot Salad 139
Corn Pasta Salad 139
Corn Relish Salad 140
Sicilian Salad 140
Sweet Sour Pasta Salad 141
Warm Shrimp Salad with Kamut 141
Zucchini Orzo Salad 142
Antipasto Pasta Salad 142
Fusilli Pasta Salad with Vegetable and Squid 143
Seashell Salad 143
Caesar Salad 144
Deli Pasta Salad With Veggies 144

Desserts and Fruits 145
Watermelon Granita 145
White Chocolate Macadamia Biscotti 145
Sicilian Chocolate Cake 146
Mediterranean fennel cakes 146
Savory Biscuits 147
Apple Strudel..........................147
Almond Italian Cookies 148
Fresh Orange Gelato 148

Panucci Fudge 148
Tiramisu Layer Cake.............149
Herbed Cheesecake..............149
Neapolitan Lemon Cookies.150
Zabaione...................................150
Italian Layer Cake 151
Poached Pears........................151
Biscotti......................................151
Italian Cheesecake.................152
Italian Rice Pudding..............152
Italian Almond Pie 153
Italian cream Hot Chocolate153
Cream Lemon Pie vanilla 154
Chocolate Salami 154
Almond Cake 155
Star Anise Biscotti..................155
Orange And Hazelnut Cake 156
Savory Tomato Pie.................156
Italian Chocolate Cake 157

21 Days Meal Plan......................158
CONCLUSION 159

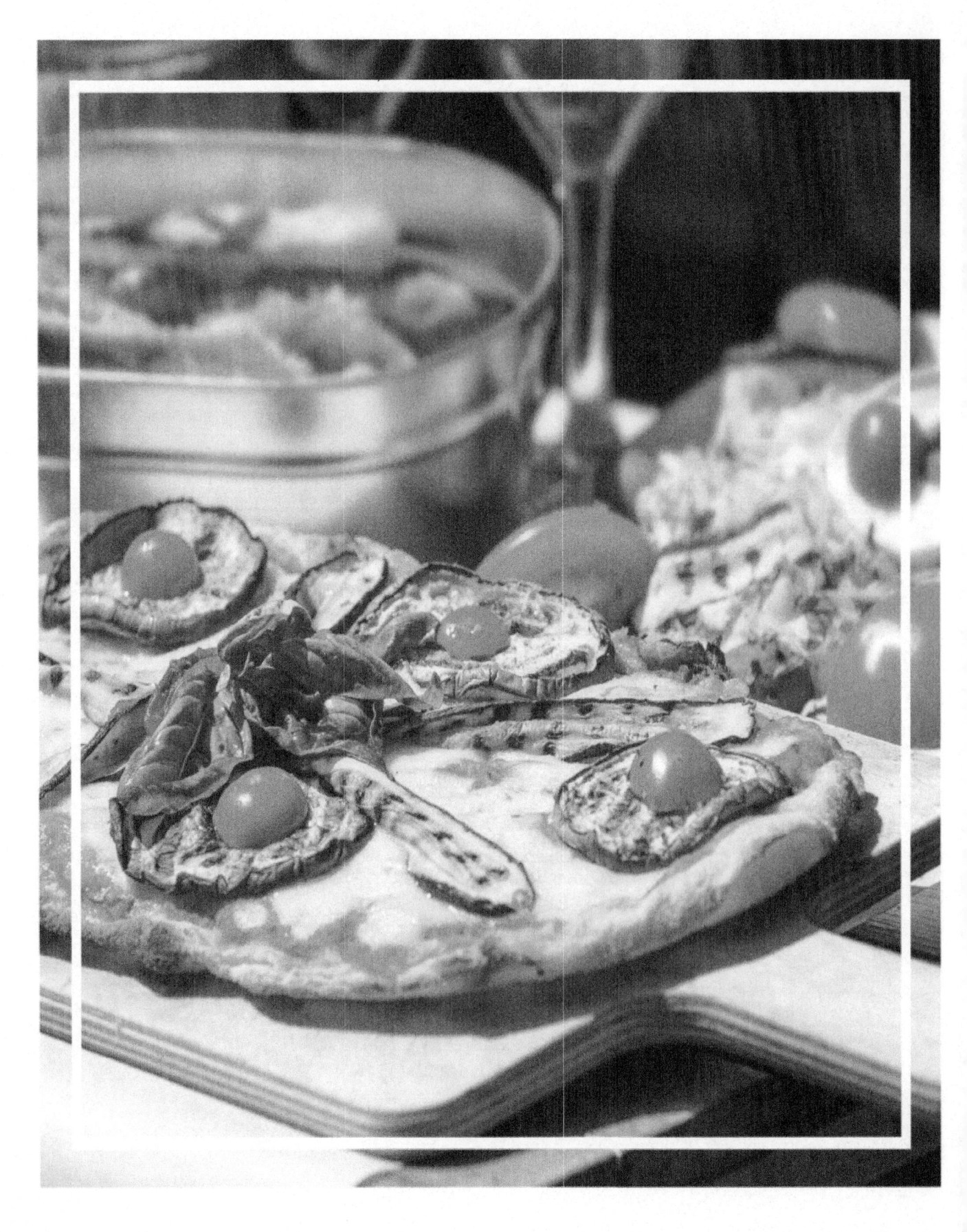

Chapter 1. Italian Cooking: Overview and History

Apparently, Italy has always been a beautiful place to live. In ancient times, it was inhabited by hunter-gatherer tribes, and then around 1000 B.C., the Etruscans emerged as an organized civilization in what is now Toscana and northern Lazio, incorporating influences from Asia Minor. They achieved farming advances like cultivated barley, lentils, and other beans (known as pulses), fruit and nuts, meat, and a custom of eating two full meals each day. They made olive oil and wine and left tombs, beautiful frescoes, and pottery, as well as writings in a language no one could translate for centuries. Meanwhile, the Phoenicians, setting sail from what is now Lebanon, settled south. To Sardegna and Sicilia, they brought exotic trade items from Egypt, possibly including dates, figs, almonds, and pomegranates. Finally, the Greeks, with their farming expertise and hunger for land, founded their first colonies on the coast of Campania. With further colonization in Sicilia and Puglia, these new colonies were used to grow wheat, olives, onions, and grapes for good wine.

Inevitably, wars broke out for land and sea routes. Some of the mercenaries who were brought in to help fight these battles decided to stay. When the Celts heard that the land was worth fighting for, they swept in, even managing at one point to get as far south as Rome before being pushed back north. Their great contribution to Italian cuisine was in their knowledge of salt: How to harvest it and how to use it to preserve food. One of their settlements was in Parma; thus, we may have them to thank for prosciutto.

Then came the Romans. Initially, the Roman diet was unsophisticated. Like the Etruscans, they made a sort of grits (puls) from ground farro and barley, now popularly called polenta. But they ate little else with it. The main meal (coena) eaten at mid-day might consist of pulses from favas and chickpeas, some vegetables, and maybe some herbs. They ate very little meat. Beef, mainly used for sacrifices, was only consumed at weddings. Food that could be stored, like cheese, was extremely precious. Only in wealthy households was there a simple approximation of an appetizer (gustaio)—maybe eggs or oysters—and then a main course containing meat. A dessert (secundae mensae) consisted of fruit or nuts. They also ate a small breakfast and a smaller dinner.

However, over the next few centuries, with the rise and expansion of the empire, things began to change. In short, the Romans learned from every people they conquered. Most important, once Hannibal and his elephants were defeated, they improved their farming and herding skills thanks to Carthaginian texts translated into Latin. With free access to all parts of Italy and its trade routes, bread, fruit, and spices appeared. And now the main meal (coena) was eaten in the evening while lunch (prandium) included leftover meat from the previous day's dinner as well as bread and cheese.

The dining excesses of the Roman wealthy are described in the first culinary writings of importance, De re coquinaria, attributed to (Marcus Garvius) Apicius. (The texts were likely compiled after he died, somewhere between the second and fourth centuries A.D.) Paradoxically, at this time, many poor Romans didn't even have a place to make a meal—living on sausages and such from tabernae (taverns). The Roman Empire generally absorbed without dictating custom. When the empire was overthrown toward the end of the fifth century, all those previously subjugated (including the tribes of native Italians, italici) were left with their different languages and cultural preferences intact. This regional individuality would be reinforced even after unification, more than a millennium later.

During the Middle Ages, parts of Italy changed hands multiple times between Byzantines and Germanic tribes—Franks, Lombards—but from the standpoint of Italian cuisine, the most important invasion occurred when the Arabs came to Sicilia in the ninth century. Besides advances in irrigation and religious tolerance, they brought pasta. As if that weren't enough, they brought, among other things, citrus trees, sugarcane, and really, the craft of making sweets.

The gradual overcoming of the classic/barbaric and the Galenic theories regarding the four bodily humors came with the Italian Renaissance. People loved hunting and agricultural products, especially local ones; rare and refined products as well as simple and natural ones; and all types of cheese and wines; sweet, strong, and simple tastes.

Arguably the most famous cooking texts of the Renaissance were written by two friends, one great cook and one iconoclastic humanist who eventually became the Vatican's librarian. Maestro Martino (Martino de Rossi, also known as Martino da Como) was the cook. He wrote a practical book for cooks in the Italian vernacular, entitled Libro de arte coquinaria. The humanist, Bartolomeo Sacchi, was known as Platina—the Latin name of the town of his birth. He took these recipes, added medical and lifestyle directives, and wrote a best-seller in elevated Latin, De honesta voluptate et valetudine (loosely translated as virtuous pleasure and good health). This book freed people from the idea that food was sinful; it spurred the growth of regional cuisines.

While those texts gave historians their best glimpse into the everyday cuisine of the Renaissance, Italians of the time were given a glimpse into the world of papal extravagance when Bartolomeo Scappi wrote Opera, which literally means "the work." Scappi was employed by several cardinals and eventually became chef to two popes. The book included precise instructions for more than a thousand recipes, as well as advice "to his apprentice" on how to set up a kitchen and menu for important occasions.

However, the elaborate banquet preparations of these times are less important than the foods that would come to Italy from the New World. To reduce their dependency on expensive imports, like spices from Asia, prosperous Spain and Portugal began to finance foreign exploration. What the explorers found and brought back to Italy would change its cuisine indelibly. Without the so-called Columbian Exchange, there would be no corn, peppers, potatoes, turkey, or tomatoes in Italy. (Interestingly, the spices that had been so in vogue when they were precious fell out of fashion when they were easier to procure.) However, these changes did not occur instantly and the Renaissance did not last forever. (At this point, we should also acknowledge the significant contribution of the Jewish communities that were present in Sicily and throughout Italy from as far back as 70 BC. With religious dietary guidelines, they adopted and adapted with the times. For example, they may have been among the first to eat eggplant in Sicily, and Carciofi alla giudia (fried artichokes) may have been invented in Rome in the 1500s as a way to replace butter in cooking.)

The 17th century was marked by recession, epidemic, and famine. And in the 18th century, the rich began to eat as the poor had all along, emphasizing simple dishes featuring local ingredients. From Italian influence and learnings, France produced over a century of great chefs and a wonderful culinary culture that also returned an influence on Italian cuisine, particularly the cuisine of the Kingdom of the Two Sicilies. Of course, this peasant food was more delicate for a newly moneyed class of landowners. The bourgeoisie also embraced coffee and chocolate, exotic ingredients that had first appeared in Venice a hundred years before.

In the 19th century, despite some powerful resistance, Italy finally became one country. During this period, France was the culinary authority in Europe (still under the lasting influence of Catherine de' Medici, who had married King Henry II and taken with her a dowry that included cooks and herbs). Unification would be a slow process, but a helping hand came in the form of a self-published cookbook. La scienza in cucina e l'arte di mangiar bene (Science in the Kitchen and the Art of Eating Well) in 1891 was the first Italian cookbook written for homemakers without servants, not elevated chefs. Its author, retired banker and silk merchant Pellegrino Artusi, began with the idea that it would be fun to ask people for recipes as he traveled around the country. The result is conversational, informative and entertaining. It is also the second most popular book ever published in Italy. Even though each region had and will always have its dishes, methods of preparation, and featured ingredients, this book provided a common language of Italian cuisine as a whole. A well-worn copy is still in most Italian households today.

During the First World War, Italy fought as one against a common enemy for the first time in its history. It also proved to be a bonding experience in taste, as men from all over the country were exposed to each other's preferences and traditions. After the war, an emphasis on modernity emerged. Practicality was also a consideration, emphasized in works such as Olindo Guerrini's L'arte di utilizzare gli avanzi della mensa (The Art of Using Leftovers) in 1917. World War II and the eventual Nazi occupation made food scarce; the food grown in the countryside was all that kept the cities fed.

So, the basic Italian tradition of eating many vegetables and grains, using olive oil and not much meat—what has become known as The Mediterranean Diet—continued as the only practical way to survive. It was only with the industrialization that began in the 1960s, which got people off of the land and into the cities, that a real threat to the old ways began to emerge.

Finally, in the late 1980s, after the experimentation of nouvelle cuisine, there was a dawning realization that the "progress" of mass-produced food, combined with continual globalization and homogenization, might not be a good thing. A single event moved concerned citizens to action: There would be a McDonald's in Rome. In response, the Slow Food Movement was born. It had the dual purpose of holding back rampant industrialization of food production and emphasizing the sensual pleasure of eating well. This concept dovetailed well with the economically driven European Union (EU) protective regulations Italy would embrace in the 1990s. Preservation of culinary traditions and financial stability could go hand in hand.

Chapter 2. The Main Ingredients in Italian Cooking

The Italian Cuisine is very diverse in nature. Each region has something unique to offer to the taster; that is why jumbling it altogether wouldn't be good for anyone or any taste buds! Italian Cuisine is a blend of fresh and diverse foods combined in a simplistic yet artistic manner that makes the food so much more than just-food. In addition, Italians don't just stuff the food as soon as it is served; they tend to enjoy it.

There are many regional variations when it comes to cooking. Still, generally, the ingredients are the same. Here are the common main ingredients used in Italian cookbook.

Grain foods:

Like other countries, grains like wheat have been the cornerstone of Italian Cuisine. But wheat is one of the most respected food as well and is not considered ordinary in any way in the Italian kitchen. Wheat is used for baking a variety of bread that includes focaccia, ciabatta, and crusty whole bread. In addition, it is used to make delicious pasta, as described in the previous chapter. There are other popular grains, too, like rice, but wheat is the king of grains in the Italian pantry.

Vegetables and fruits:

There is an ancient saying that great cooking always starts in the market and Italian food fits into this saying perfectly. There are a number of vegetables included in Italian dishes, the most popular of which are cabbage, bell peppers, tomatoes, eggplants, mushrooms, asparagus, fennel, artichokes, lettuce, and other green vegetables.

The vegetables are ordinarily chopped up and added into dishes like pasta, risottos, or pizzas. Or they are turned into salads and side dishes, which by the way, are an integral part of every Italian meal.

Coming to fruits, they are treated as post-meal snacks and included in desserts. Popular fruits include citrus fruit, berries, pears, lemons, oranges, apples, and grapes.

Olive oil:

Many of you might know of the popularity of olives and olive oil in the Italian region, especially if you've watched The Godfather! Olive is a specialty of Sothern Italy and the whole Mediterranean region in general. Olive trees are a common sight in this region, and in fact, so many olives are found that olive oil extraction is a full-blown business over here. Whole olives and olive oil are used in Italian foods like marinades, dishes, salad dressings, or as a drizzle on crusty bread.

Fish, meat, and poultry:

The Italian coastline is gifted with a variety of fish and other seafood that has become increasingly popular worldwide. Popular types include sardines, tuna, anchovies, salmon, shrimp, clamp, etc., that are added to pasta dishes, bakery items, stews, or served with olive oil.

Meat has more of a festive status in Italy and is used as a taste enhancer. Nonetheless, due to the excess of Italian festivals, plenty of dishes use meat from goats, lambs, sheep, etc.

Poultry, on the other hand, especially chicken and its eggs, is a common ingredient in the extremely popular Italian dish, frittata.

Cheeses:

France isn't the only country known for its cheeses in Europe. Italy offers a variety of options when it comes to cheeses that are eaten regularly throughout the region. Some of the most popular products in the area include Parmesan, Romano, Mozzarella, Ricotta, and Gorgonzola.

Cheeses are used to top off pizzas, pasta, risottos, salads, or virtually any dish there is.

Herbs and Seasoning:

Italians are known to enjoy the flavor of their food and are masters in bringing them out. To accomplish this feat, they use a plethora of herbs and spices like basil, rosemary, parsley, and oregano to season each dish they prepare. In addition, they also use vinegar, freshly cracked pepper, and balsamic vinegar to impart flavor to their foods.

Lemon juice is also a commonly used enhancer along with olive oil that augments the texture of many dishes like soups, pasta sauces, stews, etc. They are mainly used at the end of cooking.

Nuts:

Nuts like walnuts, almonds, and pine nuts are used in cooking and as a snack. You might know this by now, but one of Italy's most famous sauces, the pesto, is a careful mixture of garlic, basil, parmesan cheese, olive oil, and pine nuts.

Breakfast

Italian Breakfast Casseroles

Prep Time: 20 min   **Cook Time:** 40 min   **Servings:** 4

INGREDIENTS
- 4 medium red potatoes, sliced
- 2 tbsps. vegetable oil
- 8 eggs, lightly beaten
- 1 tbsp. butter
- 1/2 lb. thinly sliced fully cooked ham, diced
- 2 cups spaghetti sauce
- 1/2 cup each shredded cheddar and mozzarella cheese

DIRECTIONS
1. Fry potatoes for approximately 10-15 mins in a skillet with oil until tender; place on the bottom of 4 individual of 16-oz. dish in.
2. Scramble eggs in the same skillet with butter until set; scoop on top of the potatoes. Add ham on top. Put half cup of spaghetti sauce in each casserole; scatter with cheese.
3. Bake for 20 mins in a 350 degrees F oven or until bubbly and hot.

NUTRITION: Calories: 566 | Fat: 16g | Carbs: 34g | Protein: 34 g | Cholesterol 482 mg | Total Fat: 33 g | Fiber 4 g | Sodium: 1405 mg

Italian Mini Frittatas

Prep Time: 25 min   **Cook Time:** 50 min   **Servings:** 1

INGREDIENTS
- 2 tbsps. chopped sun-dried tomatoes (not packed in oil)
- 1/2 cup boiling water
- 2 thin slices prosciutto, finely chopped
- 1/4 cup chopped shallots
- 1 tsp. butter
- 2 garlic cloves, minced
- 1/4 cup all-purpose flour
- 1-1/2 cups fat-free milk
- 4 large egg whites
- 2 large eggs
- 1 cup shredded part-skim mozzarella cheese
- 1/4 cup shredded Asiago cheese
- 1/2 cup canned water-packed artichoke hearts, rinsed, drained and chopped
- 2 tbsps. minced fresh basil or 2 tsps. dried basil
- 3/4 tsp. salt
- 1/2 tsp. white pepper

DIRECTIONS
1. Pour boiling water over tomatoes placed in a small bowl. Cover the bowl and let sit for 5 minutes. Drain off water and set aside.
2. Sauté shallots and prosciutto in butter in a small nonstick skillet until shallots are softened. Stir in garlic, cook for 1 more minute. Turn the heat off and put to one side.
3. Combine milk and flour in a large bowl until no lumps remain; mix in the eggs and egg whites until incorporated. Mix in prosciutto mixture, reserved tomatoes, pepper, salt, basil, artichokes, and cheeses.
4. Grease 12 muffin cups using cooking spray; pour in egg mixture. Bake for 25 to 30 minutes at 350° or until an inserted knife near the middle comes out clean. Gently run a knife around the inside edges to loosen; take out of pan. Serve while warm.

NUTRITION: Calories: 172 | Fat: 11g | Protein: 15g | Total Carboydrate: 11 g | Cholesterol: 93 mg | Total Fat: 7 g | Sodium: 642 mg

Egg And Tomato Scramble

Prep Time: 5 min
Cook Time: 10 min
Servings: 1

INGREDIENTS

- 1 plum tomato, peeled and chopped
- 1 teaspoon chopped fresh basil or 1/4 teaspoon dried basil
- 1 egg or egg substitute equivalent
- 1 teaspoon water
- 1 garlic clove, minced
- 1 teaspoon olive oil, optional
- Salt and pepper to taste, optional
- 1 slice bread, toasted
- Additional fresh basil, optional

DIRECTIONS

1. Mix together basil and tomato in a small bowl; set aside. Beat garlic, water and egg in another bowl. In a small nonstick skillet, heat oil if desired; add egg mixture. Cook while stirring gently until egg is almost set. Add tomato mixture, and pepper and salt if desired.
2. Cook until egg is set completely and tomato is heated through, remember to stir while cooking. Serve with toast. Place basil on top to garnish if desired.

NUTRITION: Calories: 152 | Fat: 4g | Carbs: 20g | Protein: 11 g | Sodium: 289 mg | Cholesterol: 1 mg |

Breakfast Pizza Skillet

Prep Time: 20 min
Cook Time: 40 min
Servings: 4

INGREDIENTS

- 2/3 lb. Johnsonville® Ground Mild Italian sausage
- 3 1/3 cups frozen shredded hash brown potatoes
- 1/4 cup chopped onion
- 1/4 cup chopped green pepper
- 1/8 to 1/4 tsp. salt
- Pepper to taste
- 1/4 cup sliced mushrooms
- 3 large eggs, lightly beaten
- 1 medium tomato, thinly sliced
- 2/3 cup shredded cheddar cheese
- Sour cream and salsa, optional

DIRECTIONS

1. Cook the sausage in a prepared large pan over medium heat until it is no longer pink. Add pepper, salt, green pepper, onion, and potatoes. Cook for 18-20 minutes over medium-high heat or until the potatoes become brown.
2. Stir in mushrooms. Top the potato mixtures with eggs. Arrange sliced tomatoes on top. Top with cheese.
3. Cook, covered over medium-low heat until eggs become completely set (do not stir), or for 10-15 minutes. Serve with salsa and sour cream if preferred.

Breakfast Risotto

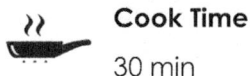

Prep Time: 15 min
Cook Time: 30 min
Servings: 4

INGREDIENTS

- 4 tbsp. (1/2 stick) butter, divided
- 4 hot Italian sausages, casings removed
- 1 small onion, chopped (about 1 cup)
- 2 small bay leaves
- 1 cup of arborio rice or medium-grain white rice
- 1/2 cup of dry white wine
- 3 cups (or more) low-salt chicken broth
- Pinch of saffron threads
- 1/3 cup chopped fresh Italian parsley
- 1/3 cup freshly grated Parmesan cheese plus additional for serving

DIRECTIONS

1. Add 2 tbsp. of the butter in a big saucepan and melt over medium-high heat.
2. Drop the sausages; break them up using a fork.
3. Stir in the following 2 ingredients.
4. Sauté for roughly 4 minutes until the onion turns translucent.
5. Mix in the rice.
6. Add wine; let the mixture boil for a minute until the liquid evaporates.
7. Stir in 3 cups of saffron and broth; let the mixture boil.
8. Adjust the heat to medium-low; make it to a simmer and stir from time to time until the risotto has softened.
9. Add an extra broth if it turns too dry, roughly 18 minutes.
10. Dispose of the bay leaves; stir in 1/3 cup of cheese and parsley.
11. Spice it up with pepper and salt.
12. Pass the cheese alongside.

NUTRITION: Calories: 100 | Fat: 6g | Carbs: 11g | Protein: 1 g

---

Italian Strata

Prep Time: 30 min
Cook Time: 1 h and 30 min
Servings: 8

INGREDIENTS

- 8 slices Italian bread
- 1 (8 oz.) ball mozzarella cheese, shredded
- 2 (14.5 oz.) cans whole tomatoes, drained and sliced
- 1 (30 oz.) can mushrooms, drained
- 1 medium onion, thinly sliced in rings
- 3 cups milk
- 5 eggs, slightly beaten
- 1 1/2 teaspoons salt
- 1/8 tablespoon garlic salt
- 1/2 teaspoon oregano
- 1/2 cup Parmesan cheese

DIRECTIONS

1. From bread, cut 8 donuts and holes. Fit the leftover scraps of cut-up bread in bottom of 13x9x2-inch greased pan. Top with a layer of cheese. Arrange tomato slices on top of cheese (reserving 8 slices for top).
2. Layer mushrooms and onion rings over cheese. Add another layer of cheese. Arrange donuts and holes and tomato slices on top of cheese. Combine milk, eggs, salt, garlic salt and oregano; pour over bread. Sprinkle with Parmesan cheese.
3. Cover with wax paper and refrigerate overnight. Remove from refrigerator 1 hour before baking. Bake at 350 degrees for 1 to 1 1/2 hours. Insert a knife in center to determine doneness. Let stand 5 minutes before cutting

Breakfast

Meatball Sandwich

Prep Time: 20 min
Cook Time: 40 min
Servings: 4

INGREDIENTS

- 1-pound ground beef
- 1 French baguette
- 3/4 cup bread crumbs
- 1 tablespoon extra-virgin olive oil
- 2 teaspoons dried Italian seasoning
- 1/2 teaspoon garlic powder
- 2 cloves garlic, minced
- 1 pinch salt, or to taste
- 2 tablespoons chopped fresh parsley
- 1 (14 ounce) jar spaghetti sauce
- 2 tablespoons grated Parmesan cheese
- 4 slices provolone cheese
- 1 egg, beaten

DIRECTIONS

1. Preheat the oven to 175 deg. Celsius (350 degrees Fahrenheit). Gently combine the bread crumbs, ground beef, Italian seasoning, garlic, parsley, Parmesan cheese, and egg in a medium mixing bowl. Form the meatballs into 12 meatballs and place them in a baking dish.
2. In a preheated oven, bake for 15 to 20 minutes, or until thoroughly done. Meanwhile, cut the baguette lengthwise in half, and remove the piece of the inside bread to make a well for the meatballs—season with garlic powder and salt after brushing with olive oil. Place the baguette in the oven for the last 5 minutes of cooking time or until gently browned.
3. With a slotted spoon, add the meatballs to the sauce after they're done. Top with provolone cheese slices and spread the mixture across the baguette. Return to the oven for about 2 1/2 minutes to melt the cheese. Allow for some cooling time before slicing into servings

NUTRITION: Calories: 781 | Fat: 31.9g | Carbs: 78.2 g | Protein: 43.6 g | Cholesterol:141 mg

---

Calico Pepper Frittata

Prep Time: 20 min
Cook Time: 30 min
Servings: 4

INGREDIENTS

- 5 large eggs
- 1-1/4 cups egg substitute
- 1 tbsp. grated Romano cheese
- 1/2 tsp. salt
- 1/8 tsp. pepper
- 1 tbsp. olive oil
- 1 medium sweet red pepper, chopped
- 1 medium green pepper, chopped
- 1 jalapeno pepper, seeded and chopped
- 1 medium onion, chopped
- 1 garlic clove, minced

DIRECTIONS

1. Beat the first 5 ingredients in a big bowl until combined.
2. On medium-high heat, heat oil in a big non-stick pan. Cook and stir onion and peppers in hot oil until tender. Put in garlic then cook for another minute. Add the egg mixture, it should set at the edges right away. Cook for 8-10mins without cover until the eggs are set completely. Push the cooked part to the middle and let the uncooked eggs flow beneath. Slice into wedges.

NUTRITION: Calories: 201 | Protein: 17 g | Total Fat: 10 g | Tot Carbohydrates: 10 g | Cholesterol; 268 mg | Fiber 2 g | Protein 17 g | Sodium: 559 mg

Egg And Tomato Scramble

Prep Time: 5 min
Cook Time: 10 min
Servings: 1

INGREDIENTS

- 3 egg
- 3 oz Parmesan
- 1/8 teaspoon salt
- 1/8 teaspoon ground white pepper
- 1/2 chili pepper
- 1 ¼ tablespoon butter
- ½ tablespoon dill
- 3 oz smoked bacon
- ½ tablespoon basil
- ½ tablespoon parsley
- 1 ½ tablespoon milk
- ½ teaspoon chili flakes
- 5 oz yeast dough
- ½ teaspoon olive oil

DIRECTIONS

1. Defrost the yeast dough.
2. Slice the smoked bacon and place it on the tray.
3. Preheat the oven to 365 F and put the tray with the sliced bacon there.
4. Pour the olive oil into the pan and preheat it.
5. Beat the eggs in the preheated olive oil and cook the eggs for 2 minutes.
6. After this, scramble the eggs. Sprinkle the eggs with the ground white pepper and add milk.
7. Mix the mixture up well and remove it from the heat.
8. Then remove the sliced bacon from the oven and chill it.
9. Then chop the sliced crunchy bacon and combine it with the scrambled egg mixture.
10. Chop the chili pepper and add it there too.
11. Then chop Parmesan and add it to the egg mixture too.
12. Separate the yeast dough into 8 medium balls and roll every ball.
13. Place the egg mixture in the middle of every ball and pinch them to make the shape of real bombs.
14. Preheat the oven to 365 F. Melt the butter and combine it with the dill, basil, parsley, and chili flakes.
15. Transfer the bombs in the round form.
16. Spread the bombs with the butter0herb mixture.
17. Out the form in the preheated oven and cook it for 30 minutes.
18. Then remove the cooked breakfast bombs from the oven and chill them for about 15 minutes.
19. Separate the breakfast bombs and serve them

NUTRITION: Calories: 368 | Fat: 21.8g | Carbs: 18.79g | Fiber: 3 g |

Breakfast Couscous

Prep Time: 15 min
Cook Time: 5 min
Servings: 4

INGREDIENTS

- ¼ cup currants, dried
- A pinch of salt
- 6 teaspoons brown sugar
- 3 cups low fat milk
- 1 cinnamon stick
- ½ cup apricots, dried and chopped
- 1 cup couscous, uncooked
- 4 teaspoons butter, melted

DIRECTIONS

1. Heat up a pan with the milk and cinnamon over medium high heat for 3 minutes and take off heat.
2. Add couscous, currants, apricots, salt and sugar, stir, cover and leave aside for 15 minutes.
3. Discard cinnamon stick, divide into bowls, sprinkle some brown sugar on top of each and serve.

NUTRITION: Calories: 250 Cal | Fat: 6.5 g | Total Carbs: 7 g | Protein: 10 g

Breakfast

Caramelized Mushroom And Onion Frittata

Prep Time: 15 min **Cook Time:** 60 min **Servings:** 4

INGREDIENTS
- 1 lb. sliced fresh mushrooms
- 1 medium red onion, chopped
- 3 tbsps. butter
- 3 tbsps. olive oil
- 1 shallot, chopped
- 1 garlic clove, minced
- 1/2 cup shredded cheddar cheese
- 1/4 cup shredded Parmesan cheese
- 8 large eggs
- 3 tbsps. heavy whipping cream
- 1/4 tsp. salt
- 1/4 tsp. pepper

DIRECTIONS
1. Add the butter and oil in a 10-in. ovenproof skillet, cook and stir the mushrooms and onion in until tender. Adjust the heat to medium-low; allow them to cook for about half an hour or until it turns deep golden brown. Stir the mixture from time to time. Stir in the garlic and shallot; let it cook for 1 minute more.
2. Lessen the heat; top it off with cheeses. Whisk the cream, eggs, pepper and salt in a big bowl; pour over top. Allow to cook for 4-6 minutes while covered or until eggs are almost set.
3. Take off the cover of the skillet. Broil, positioning the pan 3-4 in. away from the heat source for 2-3 minutes or until eggs are entirely set. Let it rest for about 5 minutes. Slice into wedges

NUTRITION: Calories: 465 | Total Fat: 38 g | Total Carbs: 11g | Protein: 22 g | Cholesterol: 479 mg | Fiber; 2 g | Sodium: 529 mg

---

Cheesy Vegetable Frittata

Prep Time: 15 min **Cook Time:** 35 min **Servings:** 4

INGREDIENTS
- 8 large eggs, beaten
- 2 cups sliced fresh mushrooms
- 1 cup chopped fresh broccoli
- 1/2 cup shredded sharp cheddar cheese
- 4 tbsps. finely chopped onion
- 4 tbsps. finely chopped green pepper
- 4 tbsps. grated Parmesan cheese
- 1/4 tsp. salt
- Dash pepper

DIRECTIONS
1. Combine all ingredients in a large bowl. Pour mixture into a shallow 2-cup baking dish coated with cooking spray.
2. Bake without a cover at 350° for 20 to 25 minutes or until a knife comes out clean when inserted in the center. Enjoy right away.

NUTRITION: Calories: 143 | Total Fat: 5 g | Total Carbs: 7 g | Protein: 19 g | Cholesterol: 14 mg | Fiber; 1 g | Sodium: 587 mg

---

Creamy Breakfast Oatmeal

Prep Time: 15 min **Cook Time:** 20 min **Servings:** 4

- ½ teaspoon cinnamon, ground
- Fresh berries for serving
- 1 cup rolled oats
- A pinch of salt
- 2 cups boiling water
- 2 teaspoons butter
- Honey for serving
- Your favorite nuts for serving

1. Put boiling water in a pan, add oats, bring to a boil over medium heat, cook for 5 minutes, reduce heat and cook for 10 more minutes string all the time.
2. Take pot off the heat, add cinnamon and butter, cover and leave aside for 5 minutes.
3. Stir oats again, divide into bowls, top with berries, honey and nuts and serve.

NUTRITION: Calories: 160 Cal | Fat: 3 g | Carbs: 30 g | Protein: 6 g

Chicken 'n' Ham Frittata

Prep Time: 15 min
Cook Time: 30 min
Servings: 6

INGREDIENTS

- 1/2 cup chopped green onions
- 2 garlic cloves, minced
- 2 tbsps. canola oil
- 1-1/4 cups chopped yellow summer squash
- 1 cup chopped zucchini
- 1/2 cup chopped sweet yellow pepper
- 1/2 cup chopped sweet red pepper
- 1 tsp. minced fresh gingerroot
- 2 cups cubed cooked chicken breast
- 1 cup chopped deli ham
- 6 large eggs
- 3/4 cup mayonnaise
- 1/4 tsp. prepared horseradish
- 1/4 tsp. pepper
- 1 cup shredded Monterey Jack cheese

DIRECTIONS

1. In a large ovenproof skillet, sauté the garlic and onions in oil, 1 minute. Include in ginger, peppers, zucchini and yellow squash; cook while stirring till vegetables are crispy-tender, or for 8 minutes. Include in ham and chicken; cook for 1 more minute or till heated through. Take away from the heat.
2. In a large bowl, beat pepper, horseradish, mayonnaise and eggs till blended. Pour into the skillet.
3. Bake without a cover at 350° till eggs are totally set, or for 25-30 minutes. Top with cheese; cover and let stand till the cheese is melted, or for 5 minutes.

NUTRITION: Calories: 504 | Total Fat: 40 g | Total Carbs: 5 g | Protein: 30 g | Cholesterol: 286 mg | Fiber; 1 g | Sodium: 669 mg

Ricotta Pancakes

Prep Time: 20 min
Cook Time: 15 min
Servings: 4

INGREDIENTS

- ½ teaspoon baking soda
- 1/8 teaspoon salt
- 1 tablespoon olive oil
- ½ teaspoon vanilla extract
- ½ teaspoon cinnamon
- 2 eggs
- 3 oz flour
- 1 ½ tablespoon brown sugar
- ½ cup ricotta cheese

DIRECTIONS

1. Crack the eggs into the mixer bowl and whisk them.
2. After this, add ricotta cheese and mix the mixture up with the help of the wooden spatula.
3. Sift the flour and add salt.
4. After this, add brown sugar and baking soda.
5. Then sprinkle the pancake mix with the vanilla extract and cinnamon, and add 1 tablespoon olive oil.
6. Take the hand mixer and mix the dough until it has the texture of the smooth sour cream.
7. Place the cooked dough in the fridge for 10 minutes.
8. Meanwhile, spray the pan with the 1 tablespoon of olive oil inside and preheat it on the medium heat.
9. Then remove the dough from the fridge and ladle the medium amount of the dough in the preheated pan.
10. Make the pancake and cook it for 3 minutes from the one side.
11. After this, turn the pancake to another side and cook it for 1.5 minutes more.
12. Make the same steps with all the dough.
13. Serve the prepared dish immediately.

NUTRITION: Calories: 221 | Total Fat: 11.2 g | Carbs: 20.08 g | Protein: 9 g | Fiber; 1 g |

Breakfast

Italian Brunch Torte

Prep Time: 50 min
Cook Time: 1 h and 50 min
Servings: 4

INGREDIENTS

- 2/3 tubes (8 oz. each) refrigerated crescent rolls, divided
- 1/3 tsp. olive oil
- 1/3 package (6 oz.) fresh baby spinach
- 1/3 cup sliced fresh mushrooms
- 3 medium eggs
- 1/3 cup grated Parmesan cheese
- 2/3 tsps. Italian seasoning
- 1/16 tsp. pepper
- 1/6 lb. thinly sliced deli ham
- 1/6 lb. thinly sliced hard salami
- 1/6 lb. sliced provolone cheese
- 2/3 jars (12 oz. each) roasted sweet red peppers, drained, sliced and patted dry

DIRECTIONS

1. Set the oven to 350° and start preheating. Grease a 9-in. springform pan and place it on a heavy-duty foil (about 18 in. square) with double thickness. Securely wrap the pan with foil. Unroll and separate 1 tube of crescent dough into triangles. To create a crust, press onto bottom of prepared pan, seal seams well. Bake until set or for 10-15 minutes.
2. In the meantime, heat oil over medium-high heat in a large skillet. Add mushrooms and spinach; cook while stirring until mushrooms become tender. Drain on several layers of paper towels, blot well. Beat pepper, Italian seasoning, Parmesan cheese and 6 eggs in a large bowl.
3. Layer crust with 1/2 each of ham, salami, provolone cheese, red peppers and spinach mixture. Pour 1/2 of the egg mixture over top. Repeat layers, place the remaining egg mixture on top.
4. On a work surface, unroll the remaining crescent dough and divide them into triangles. Press together to shape a circle, seal seams; put over filling. Beat remaining eggs and brush over dough.
5. Bake without a cover until a thermometer reads 160° or for 1 to 1-1/4 hours, loosely cover with foil if necessary to prevent overbrowning. Using a knife, loosen sides from pan carefully; remove the rim from the pan. Allow to sit for 20 minutes.

NUTRITION: Calories: 403 | Total Fat: 24 g | Total Carbs: 19g | Protein: 23 g | Cholesterol: 167 mg | Fiber: 0 g | Sodium: 1360 mg

Simple Italian Omelete

Prep Time: 10 min
Cook Time: 5 min
Servings: 1

INGREDIENTS

- 2 tablespoons olive oil
- 3 large eggs, beaten
- 1 tbsp. crumbled goat cheese
- 2 teaspoons chopped chives
- a pinch of sea salt
- ground black pepper to taste
-

DIRECTIONS

1. In a large pan, heat the olive oil over medium heat, moving it around to coat the pan. Pour eggs onto a heated skillet; they will quickly bubble and harden up.
2.
3. Lift the cooked sides of the omelet with a rubber spatula and tilt the skillet so the uncooked egg runs below. Cook, lifting the sides and flipping the skillet as needed, until the omelet is almost set for about 2 minutes. Remove from heat. Spread any runny egg on top of the omelet evenly using a spatula.
4.
5. Over the omelet, sprinkle goat cheese, 1 1/2 teaspoons chives, sea salt, and black pepper. Fold one third of the omelet into the middle, carefully lifting one side over the cheese and chives, and fold the remaining 1/3 into the center. Fold the opposite third of the omelet into the middle. Slide the omelet to the edge of the skillet and set it on a plate, folded side down. Finish with the remaining chives.

NUTRITION: Calories: 479.5 | Total Fat: 44 g | Carbs: 1.4 g | Protein: 20.5 g | Sodium: 567 mg

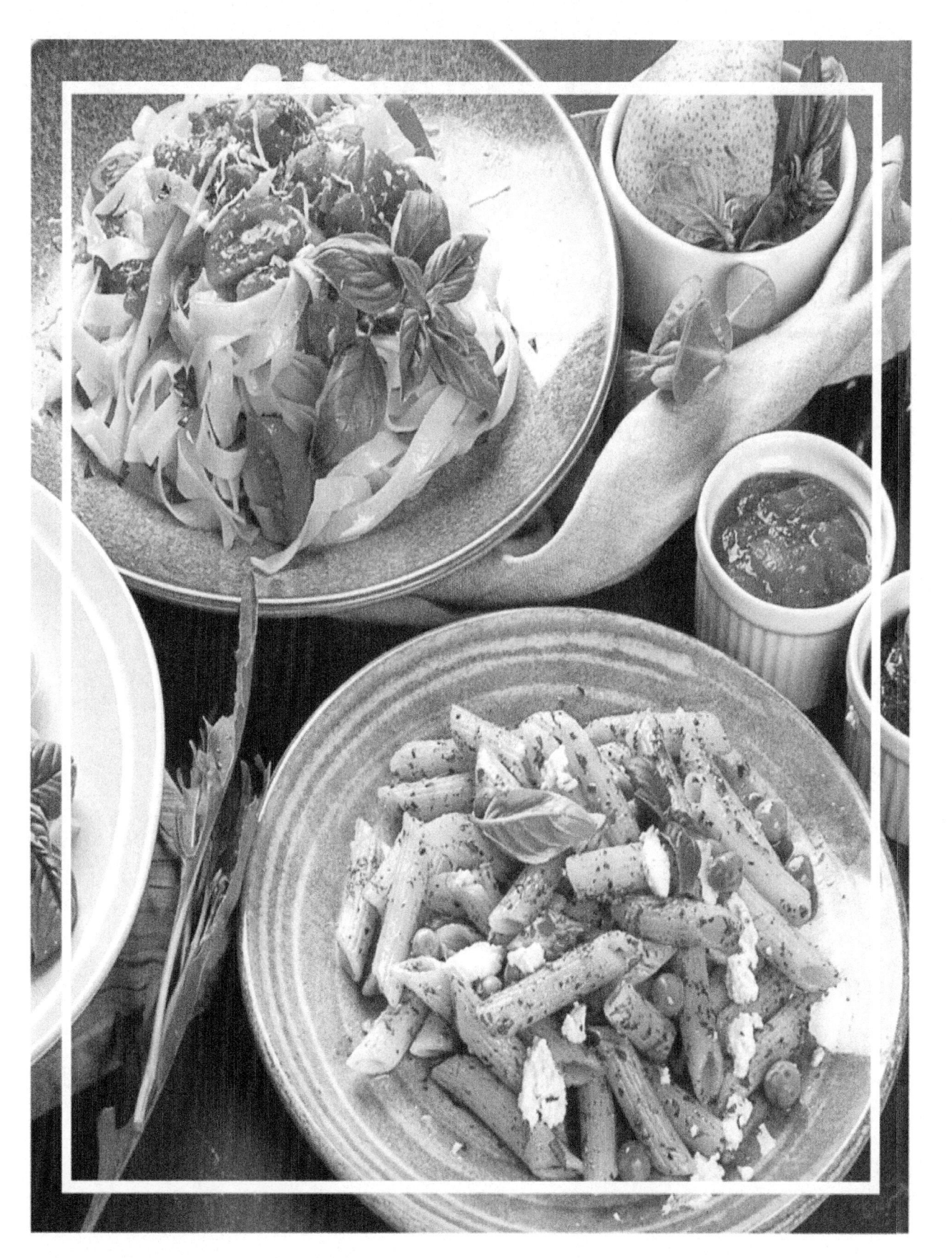

Pasta

Penne Pasta with Spinach and Bacon

Prep Time 10 min **Cook Time** 15 min **Servings** 4

INGREDIENTS

- 1 (12 ounce) package penne pasta
- 2 tablespoons minced garlic
- 2 tablespoons olive oil, divided
- 1 (14.5 ounce) can diced tomatoes
- 6 slices bacon, chopped
- 345 grams fresh spinach, torn into bite-size pieces

DIRECTIONS

1. A big saucepan of lightly salted water should be brought to a boil— Cook for 10 minutes, or until the penne pasta is soft.
2. Heat 1 tablespoon of olive oil in a separate skillet over medium heat. Cook the bacon until brown and crisp. Cook for another minute after adding the garlic. Cook, constantly stirring, until the tomatoes are cooked through.
3. Place the spinach in a colander and pour boiling water over it to wilt it. Toss with the olive oil, bacon, and tomato mixture in a large serving bowl.

NUTRITION: Calories: 517 | Fat: 16g | Carbs: 73.8g | Protein: 21 g | Cholesterol 15 mg |

Pasta with Lentils

Prep Time 25 min **Cook Time** 50 min **Servings** 1

INGREDIENTS

- 8 tablespoons Olive Oil
- 8 ounce dry Lentils
- 1 medium Onion, minced
- 2 stalks Celery, minced
- 5 cloves Garlic, minced
- 1 cup chopped San Marzano Plum Tomatoes
- 2 Chicken Bullion Cubes (optional)
- 1 Bay Leaf
- 1 –10 ounce package frozen spinach, thawed
- 1 lb. Pasta Gemmeli, Small Shells, or Fusilli
- grated Pecorino Romano, Parmigiano, or Grana

DIRECTIONS

1. In a big 6 quart pot, combine 14 cup olive oil and onions. Cook for 5 minutes on low heat, stirring regularly. Add celery and cook for another 5 minutes. Cook for 2 minutes after adding the red pepper and garlic.
2. Cook for 4 minutes on high heat with the tomatoes. Cook for 3 minutes, stirring constantly with a wooden spoon. Add bay leaf and add water ennough to cover the lentils by one inch. Cook, stirring occasionally, until lentils are cooked but still firm, about 22 minutes.
3. Chop the thawed spinach and add it to the lentils. Cook over medium heat for 5 minutes.
4. Cook the pasta according to the intructions in the package. Drain onto a colander when done, saving a few tablespoons of water to toss with the pasta.
5. Drizzle some Olive Oil over the drained pasta and return it to the saucepan it was cooked in. Add lentils to the past and mix with a big slotted spoon.
6. Add a little of the pasta cooking water if needed. You don't want the spaghetti to be too wet, but it should be slightly slack. To do so, add little amounts of liquid at a time until you attain the desired consistency.
7. Drizzle with a little more olive oil and sprinkle with grated cheese before serving.

White Lasagna with mushrooms

Prep Time: 5 min
Cook Time: 10 min
Servings: 1

INGREDIENTS

- 1/4 cup of white wine
- salt and pepper, for taste
- 1 tbsp. of freshly chopped rosemary
- 1 tbsp. of newly cut oregano
- 1 tbsp. of freshly chopped thyme
- 2 tbsp. of olive oil
- 2 spicy Italian sausages, casings removed
- 2 cups of mushrooms, thinly sliced
- 4 tbsp. of butter
- 2 cups of whole milk
- pinch of cayenne pepper
- pinch of nutmeg
- ½ lb. of lasagna noodles, cooked
- 1 onion, finely chopped
- 3 cloves of garlic, finely chopped
- 1/4 cup of flour
- 1/2 cup of thinly sliced mozzarella cheese
- half cup of grated Parmesan cheese

DIRECTIONS

1. Take a large skillet and heat the olive oil over medium heat. Then add sausage and fry until done by crushing it into small pieces with a spatula.
2. Then add mushrooms and cook until tender for four to five minutes. Cook until the liquid has entirely evaporated after deglazing the pan with wine. —season with salt, pepper, and herbs and reserve the mixture.
3. Take a middle pan and thaw the butter over medium heat. Then garlic and sauté for another minute until fragrant.
4. Stir in the flour and cook for a few more minutes. Slowly whisk in the milk, then whisk continuously until there are no more lumps.
5. Heat béchamel until thick enough to cover the back of the spoon. Season with pepper, nutmeg, salt, and cayenne pepper. Exterminate the fire and stay aside.
6. Start by layering the noodles in a separate loaf pan or small frying pan. Next, spread a layer of béchamel over the noodles and cover it with the layer of the sausage mushroom mixture.
7. Do it again until the fillings and noodles are used and finish with the layer of béchamel on the top part.
8. Top with shredded cheese. Bake lasagna until cheese is golden and sausage is bubbly for 20 to 30 minutes.

Spaghetti Picchi Pacchiu

Prep Time: 25 min
Cook Time: 50 min
Servings: 1

INGREDIENTS

- 1 pint ripe Cherry Tomatoes, washed and cut in half
- 1/3 cup Olive Oil
- 5 Garlic Cloves, peeled an sliced thin
- ½ teaspoon of Peperoncino (Red Pepper flakes)
- ½ teaspoon Sicilian Sea Salt
- ¼ cup fresh torn Basil Leaves

DIRECTIONS

1. Place the garlic and olive oil in a pan and cook on low heat for 3 minutes. Add Red Pepper Flakes and Tomatoes and cook on high heat for 6-7 minutes while stirring with a wooden spoon. Add Basil and cook on low heat 1 minute. Turn heat off and let set.
2. Cook the spaghetti in boiling salted water according to directions on package. When done, drain, reserving about 5 tablespoons of the pasta cooking water.
3. Add the drained spaghetti and reserved pasta water to pan with tomatoes and olive oil and mix.
4. Plate spaghetti onto 4 plates and serve. Eat as is, or sprinkle a little Pecorino Romano Cheese on top.

Baked Ziti

Prep Time: 30 min
Cook Time: 1 hour
Servings: 12

INGREDIENTS

- 1 pound dry ziti pasta
- 1 1/2 (26 ounce) jars spaghetti sauce
- 1 1/2 tablespoons olive oil
- salt to taste
- 1 onion, sliced
- 1 (6 ounce) package provolone cheese, sliced
- 1 teaspoon minced fresh rosemary
- 3/4 cup sour cream
- 4 cloves garlic, chopped
- 3/4 cup cottage cheese
- 1/2 pound ground beef
- 1 (6 ounce) package mozzarella cheese, shredded
- 1/2 pound ground pork sausage
- 2 tablespoons freshly grated Parmesan cheese

DIRECTIONS

1. Bring a pot of lightly salted water to a boil. Cook pasta for 8 - 10 mins in boiling water, or until al dente; drain.
2. Meanwhile, in a big, heavy skillet, heat the olive oil over medium heat. Cook the onion in the oil until it is soft. Add the garlic and rosemary and mix well. Place in a small bowl.
3. In a skillet, combine the ground meat and sausage. Cook until uniformly browned over medium-high heat. Combine the onion mixture and the spaghetti sauce in a mixing bowl. Season with salt and pepper. Lower the heat and cook for 10 minutes more.
4. Preheat oven to 350 degrees F (175 degrees C). Grease a 9x13 inch baking dish. In the prepared dish, layer 1/2 of the cooked pasta, provolone cheese, sour cream, cottage cheese, and a little less than 1/2 of the meat mixture. Then layer the rest of the pasta, mozzarella cheese, remaining meat mixture, and Parmesan cheese.
5. Bake in the oven for 20-30 min, or until heated through and cheeses are melted.

NUTRITION: Calories: 489 | Fat: 24.5g | Carbs: 43.8g | Protein: 22.1 g | Cholesterol: 55mg

Spaghetti With Clams

Prep Time: 8 min
Cook Time: 20 min
Servings: 4

INGREDIENTS

- 12 oz. (350 g) spaghetti.
- 2 1/4 lbs. (1 kg) clams, rubbed.
- 6 3/4 tbsp. (100 ml) extra-virgin olive oil.
- 1 tbsp. sliced fresh parsley.
- 1 clove garlic, cut.
- Salt and pepper.

DIRECTIONS

1. Bring a pot of well-salted water to a boil.
2. Warmth 1 tablespoon. Of oil in a huge frying pan. Include clams, cover, and chef up until they open up, 2-3 minutes get rid of frying pan from warm. Get rid of a few of clams from their coverings, pressure cooking liquid, and afterwards pour it back into skillet with clams. Allotted.
3. In another skillet, warmth continuing to be oil until hot. Include garlic and also chef till browned. Add clams and also their liquid as well as give a boil.
4. Meanwhile, prepare spaghetti in boiling water up until al dente. Drainpipe, scheduling some of pasta water. Include pasta to calm combination, adding a little pasta water if you want a wetter dish. Transfer to pasta bowls as well as serve, sprayed generously with pepper and also parsley.

Italian Cookbook 2022

Artichoke Spinach Lasagna

Prep Time: 20 min **Cook Time:** 1 hour **Servings:** 8

INGREDIENTS

- Cooking spray
- 1 (14 ounce) can marinated artichoke hearts, drained and chopped
- 9 uncooked lasagna noodles
- 1 (10 ounce) package frozen chopped spinach, thawed, drained and squeezed dry
- 1 onion, chopped
- 1 (28 ounce) jar tomato pasta sauce
- 4 cloves garlic, chopped
- 3 cups shredded mozzarella cheese, divided
- 1 (4 ounce) package herb and garlic feta
- 1 (14.5 ounce) can vegetable broth
- 1 tbsp. fresh rosemary, chopped

DIRECTIONS

1. Preheat the oven to 350 degrees Fahrenheit (180 degrees Celsius). Using cooking spray, coat a 9x13-inch baking dish.
2. Bring a saucepan of salted water to a boil. Cook, stirring occasionally, until the noodles are al dente, about 8 to 10 minutes.
3. Cook on medium-high in a large skillet sprayed with cooking spray. 3 minutes, or until onion is tender-crisp, sauté onion and garlic. Bring to a boil with the broth and rosemary. Reduce heat to low, cover, and cook for 5 minutes after adding the artichoke hearts and spinach. Add the pasta sauce and mix well.
4. Spread a fourth of the artichoke mixture on the top of the baking pan; then top with 3 cooked noodles. Over the noodles, sprinkle 3/4 cup mozzarella cheese. Layer the artichoke mixture and mozzarella cheese two more times, finishing with the artichoke mixture and mozzarella cheese. Top with crumbled feta cheese.
5. Cover and bake for 40 minutes. Remove the lid. Bake for another 17 minutes, or until it bubbles. Allow for a 10-minute rest before cutting.

NUTRITION: Calories: 369 | Fat: 16 g | Carbs: 44 g | Protein: 21.1 g | Cholesterol: 42 g

Pasta with Zucchini and Shrimp

Prep Time: 10 min **Cook Time:** 24 min **Servings:** 4

INGREDIENTS

- 320 g semolina pasta, durum wheat
- Extra virgin olive oil
- 1 garlic clove
- 2 courgettes
- ½ white wine glass
- 200 g shelled shrimps
- 1 sprig Parsley
- 1 onion

DIRECTIONS

1. Wash the onion and chop them into rings. Wash the courgettes and slice them. In running tap water, wash the peeled shrimp. Cut the garlic clove into two and chop one piece. Wash the parsley and chop them too and put them together with the garlic.
2. Make the dressing: add 2 tbsp virgin oil to a nonstick pan and add in the onion. Fry them for about 2 minutes and then add in the courgettes. Sauté for about 9 minutes. Pour in the shrimp, salt and stir. Add some white wine and cook for about 9 minutes.
3. Prepare the pasta. Add salted water to a pot and bring to boil. Add in the pasta and cook al dente as per the package instructions.
4. Drain the pasta and put it in a pan with the shrimps and courgettes. Cook for about 3-4 minutes while constantly stirring. Turn the heat off and finish with the recipe. Serve and enjoy.

Pasta

Vegetarian Cabbage Rolls

Prep Time 20 min
Cook Time 30 min
Servings 8

INGREDIENTS

- 1/3 cup uncooked brown rice
- 2/3 cup water
- 2 cups textured vegetable protein
- 3/4 cup boiling water
- 2 (10.75-oz) cans tomato soup
- 10 3/4 fluid oz. water
- 2 pinches cayenne pepper
- 1 large head cabbage, cored
- 1/2 tsp. onion powder
- 1 tbsp. vegetable oil
- 1 egg, lightly beaten
- 1 large onion, chopped
- 1/2 carrot, finely chopped
- 3 drops hot red pepper sauce
- 1/2 red bell pepper, diced
- 3 cloves garlic, minced
- salt and pepper to taste
- 1 tbsp. white wine
- 1/2 cup frozen peas
- 1 tsp. garlic powder
- 1/2 tsp. dried basil
- 1 (14.5-oz) can of whole peeled tomatoes

DIRECTIONS

1. In a pot, put 2/3 cup of water and the rice, then set to a boil. Lower heat to low, simmer while covered for about 40 minutes until tender. In a medium bowl, blend 3/4 cup of boiling water and the textured vegetable protein. Soak for 15 minutes until rehydrated. Stir in the cooked rice.
2. Preheat oven to 350° F (175° C). Stir 10 and 3/4 fluid oz. of (1 soup can) water and tomato soup in a bowl.
3. In a pot, put the cabbage and enough water to cover. Boil, then cook for 15 minutes till leaves can be removed with ease. Drain, cool, then separate the leaves.
4. In a frying pan, heat the oil over medium heat—mix in the garlic, red bell pepper, carrot, and onion. Cook until softened. Blend in wine, and keep cooking till most of the liquid has evaporated. Mix in textured vegetable protein and rice, reserved juice from tomatoes, peas, and egg. Flavor with hot pepper sauce, basil, garlic powder, onion powder, and cayenne pepper. Cook and whisk till heated through.
5. On a cabbage leaf, position 1 tomato, and 2 tbsps. Of skillet mixture. Roll firmly, then secure using a toothpick. Do the same with the leftover filling—line in a casserole dish. Spread water and soup over cabbage rolls—spice with pepper and salt.
6. In the preheated oven, bake, covered, for 35 minutes while infrequently basting with the tomato sauce. Take off the cover, and go on baking for 10 minutes.

Vermicelli With Tomato Sauce

Prep Time 30 min
Cook Time 15 min
Servings 4

INGREDIENTS

- 10 1/2 oz. (300 g).
- Vermicelli or bucatini 5 oz. (150 g) bacon or.
- guanciale, cut in tiny pieces.
- 3 1/2 tbsp. (50 ml) added virgin olive oil.
- 1 1/2 oz. (40 g) Pecorino Romano, grated, or concerning 1/2 cup.
- 1 red chile, sliced.
- Salt and pepper.

DIRECTIONS

1. Warmth oil in a skillet up until hot. Include onion as well as garlic and chef up until golden brownish. Include tomatoes, period with Salt and pepper, and continue to cook over a high warmth for around 20 minutes, stirring sometimes. Get rid of garlic as well as mix in basil.
2. Bring a pot of well-salted water to a boil. Cook pasta in boiling water until al dente and drainpipe. Transfer to bowls, put Sauce over pasta, and offer.

Classic Baked Pasta

Prep Time: 30 min
Cook Time: 1 h and 20 min
Servings: 10

INGREDIENTS

For baked pasta
- 600 g Rigatoni
- 3 tbsp Parmesan cheese DOP to grate
- 300 g Scamorza provola
- 4 Medium eggs

For the meatballs
- 250 g Ground pork
- 100 g Parmesan cheese DOP to be grated
- 2 tbsp Chopped parsley
- 150 g Sausage
- Salt to taste
- 100 g Bread crumbs
- 2 Medium eggs
- 1 pinch Nutmeg
- Black pepper to taste

For the sauce
- Tomato sauce
- 4 tbsp Extra virgin olive oil
- Salt to taste
- 1 White onions
- 5 Basil leaves
- Black pepper to taste
- 1 Garlic clove

For the bechamel
- 80 g 00 flour
- 80 g Butter
- 1 l Whole milk
- 1 pinch Nutmeg
- Salt to taste

DIRECTIONS

1. For pasta preparing in the oven, begin with the meatball's dough. Begin by taking the sausage and cutting it in half to remove the casing with surrounds it. Use a knife to chop the meat roughly.
2. Pour the minced meat in a large bowl and add the grated parmesan, chopped parsley, sausage and the breadcrumbs that were previously crumbled in a mixer.
3. Season with pepper and salt after adding the eggs. Use your hands to work on the dough until you get a homogeneous mixture. Use a plastic wrap to cover it and leave it to rest until the meatballs are prepared.
4. Now take care of the sauce. Pour the finely chopped onions, whole garlic clove and oil in a large non-stick pan. Once the oil is hot, pour in the salt, pepper and tomato puree and on low heat, cover with a lid and cook for 30 minutes occasionally stirring.
5. Meanwhile, shape meatballs of 10 g each and put them on a plate. With this amount of dough, you can get like 70 meatballs. Remove the garlic and pour the meatballs in the sauce after its cooking time is over.
6. Use pepper and salt to season and then use a spatula to mix. Over low heat, allow it to cook for 15 minutes. Add the chopped basil leaves and leave to cook for more 5 minutes.
7. Lastly, go to eggs preparation. Boil them for 10 minutes to firm them after boiling water. Under running water, cool them. Shell the hard-boiled eggs once they are cold and using a sharp knife or any other appropriate tool, cut them in slices and keep them in a small bowl aside.
8. Cut the scamorza into slice and then into strips and lastly into cubes. Set them aside after putting them in a small bowl.
9. Now go to the preparation of the bechamel. In a saucepan, heat the milk. On low heat, heat the butter into small pieces and allow it to melt in a separate pan. To the flour, add the melted butter after turning off the heat. Use a hand whisk to stir in order to avoid lumps vigorously.
10. Take the saucepan back to the heat and over low heat, cook the obtained cream until it becomes golden. You will then get a roux. Using a wire, add the hot milk and use salt and nutmeg to season.
11. On low heat, cook the bechamel for 5-6 minutes until it becomes thick. Continue mixing using a hand whisk. You can now transfer the bechamel to a bowl and then use a cling film to cover it until the time it will be used. This helps avoiding crust formation on the surface.
12. In much salted water, boil the pasta and through cooking, drain it half way. Get the ready-made meatball sauce and add it to the pasta. Use a spoon to mix the ingredients well and on the bottom, of a baking dish distribute a bechamel layer and create the first layer of meatballs and rigatoni.
13. Over the dough, spread half of the diced scamorza and half the sliced boiled eggs and use half of the grated parmesan to sprinkle.
14. Use a few spoonfuls of bechamel to season the first layer and continue to the second layer of meatballs and pasta evenly distributing it over the first one. Use other sliced eggs distributed evenly on the baking dish to complete the layer.
15. Use bechamel and diced scamorza to sprinkle. Use the remaining grated parmesan to sprinkle and over a static oven bake at 180 degrees for 15 minutes.
16. Set the oven function to grill mode after cooking and cook au gratin for 5 minutes. The basked pasta is now ready. Allow it to rest for 5-10 minutes at room temperature before you enjoy it.

Pasta

Milanese Risotto

Prep Time 30 min | **Cook Time** 20 min | **Servings** 6

- 11 1/2 oz. (320 g) Arborio rice.
- 1/4 mug (60 ml) extra-virgin olive oil.
- 8-10 small crabs, cut into quarters 5 cups (1.2 l) warm fish supply.
- 3 1/2 tablespoon. (50 ml) white wine.
- 3 1/2 oz. (100 g) squash blooms, cleaned up and also washed.
- 1/2 tbsp. (10 g) grated.
- Pecorino Romano.
- 1/2 tablespoon. (15 g) grated.
- Parmigiano-Reggiano.
- 1/3 cup plus 1 1/2 tbsp. (100 ml) extra-virgin olive oil.
- 1 tablespoon. ache nuts.
- 1/4 clove garlic.
- 1 tablespoon. diced fresh parsley Salt and pepper

1. In a Saucepan or Dutch oven, thaw fifty percent of butter over medium warmth. Add onion as well as cook till softened. Stir in rice and chef carefully For 1 minute. Pour in gewürztraminer, enable it to vaporize. Add stock in increments and continue to prepare. 5 minutes prior to rice has actually finished Food preparation, include saffron as well as period with Salt and pepper.
2. When all fluid has actually been absorbed by rice, but when it is still al dente, get rid of from heat. Whisk in remaining butter and also Parmigiano-Reggiano.

Pasta Fagioli

Prep Time 10 min | **Cook Time** 40 min | **Servings** 4

- 1 tablespoon olive oil
- salt to taste
- 2 stalks celery, chopped
- 1 (14.5 ounce) can chicken broth
- 1 onion, chopped
- 2 medium tomatoes, peeled and chopped
- 3 cloves garlic, minced
- 1 (8 ounce) can tomato sauce
- 2 teaspoons dried parsley
- 1/2 cup uncooked spinach pasta
- 1 teaspoon Italian seasoning
- 1 (15 ounce) can cannellini beans, with liquid
- 1/4 teaspoon crushed red pepper flakes

1. Heat the olive oil in the medium in a large saucepan. When hot, cook celery, onion, garlic, parsley, Italian seasoning, red pepper flakes, and salt until onion is translucent.It takes 5 minutes.
2. Simmer on low for 16 to 20 minutes after adding the chicken stock, tomatoes, and tomato sauce.
3. Cook until pasta is tender. Add undrained beans and mix well. Bring to a boil.
4. Serve with grated Parmesan cheese on top.

Spaghetti with Garlic Sauce

Prep Time 15 min | **Cook Time** 20 min | **Servings** 4

- 1 lb. spaghetti, cooked
- 1/2 cup butter
- 1/2 cup extra-virgin olive oil
- 4 small cloves garlic, minced
- 2 tablespoons fresh parsley, chopped
- Parmesan cheese, grated

1. Cook pasta according to package directions; drain and set aside.
2. Meanwhile, melt butter in a large pan. Add olive oil. Sauté minced garlic in oil until golden brown. Add cooked spaghetti and parsley. Cook over low heat until heated through. Serve with grated Parmesan cheese.

Spaghetti with Clam Sauce

Prep Time 10 min **Cook Time** 15 min **Servings** 4

- 3 tablespoons olive oil, plus more for drizzling
- 1 garlic clove, minced
- ½ teaspoon salt
- 25 to 30 clams, scrubbed clean
- ½ cup dry white wine (see wine pairing tip)
- 12 ounces spaghetti
- 1 tablespoon chopped fresh parsley

1. In a large sauté pan over medium-high heat, heat the oil and garlic for about 1 minute. Add the salt, clams, and wine, cover, and cook for 5 minutes. Discard any unopened clams.
2. Meanwhile, cook the spaghetti in boiling salted water for 1 to 2 minutes less than directed on the package.
3. Drain the spaghetti and add to the pan with the clams. Finish cooking for an additional minute or two, or until the spaghetti is al dente. Transfer the pasta to a large serving bowl and sprinkle with the parsley. Top with an additional drizzle of oil, if desired.

Spaghetti with Tomato Sauce

Prep Time 15 min **Cook Time** 30 min **Servings** 4

- 2 tablespoons extra-virgin olive oil
- 1 large onion, finely chopped
- 1 clove garlic, finely chopped
- 1 (28 oz.) can whole San Marzano Italian tomatoes, undrained
- 1 (6 oz.) can tomato paste
- 1 bay leaf
- 1 teaspoon basil
- 1 teaspoon oregano
- Salt and pepper to taste
- 12 oz. spaghetti

1. Heat olive oil in a medium saucepan. Add onion and garlic; sauté until onion is translucent. Add tomatoes, tomato paste, bay leaf, basil, oregano, salt and pepper. Bring to a boil; simmer for 30 minutes.
2. Cook spaghetti in boiling, salted water following package directions; drain. Place spaghetti in heated serving bowl. Pour tomato sauce on top, and serve.

Veal Cutlets with Tomato and Basil Sauce

Prep Time 15 min **Cook Time** 20-30 min **Servings** 6

- 8 oz. bow tie pasta, cooked as package directs and drained
- 2 tablespoons flour
- 1 tablespoon freshly grated Parmesan cheese
- 1/8 teaspoon pepper
- 3/4 lb. veal cutlets, sliced 1/8 inch thick
- 2 tablespoons extra-virgin olive oil
- 1 (26 oz.) jar Tomato Basil Pasta Sauce
- 1/2 cup (2 oz.) shredded mozzarella cheese

1. In a shallow dish, combine flour, Parmesan cheese and pepper. Dip meat into flour mixture, coating both sides. In a large skillet, over medium heat, cook meat in olive oil for 2 minutes or until light brown, turning once. Remove meat from pan, reserving drippings in skillet. Set meat aside.
2. Add pasta sauce to skillet. Bring to a boil; reduce heat. Cover; simmer for 5 minutes. Return meat to skillet; heat through. Serve over hot bow tie pasta. Sprinkle with mozzarella cheese.

Pasta

Sicilian Eggplant Rigatoni

Prep Time: 1 hour
Cook Time: 10 min
Servings: 4

INGREDIENTS

- 12 oz. (350 g) rigatoni.
- 9 oz. (250 g) eggplant.
- 2 tbsp. (30 ml) extra-virgin olive oil.
- 2 oz. (50 g) yellow onion, about sliced 1 clove garlic.
- 2 lbs. (1 kg) ripe tomatoes, diced 6 leaves fresh basil.
- 2 oz. (50 g) grated ricotta salata, or concerning 1/2 mug.
- Salt and pepper flour as required

DIRECTIONS

1. In a skillet, warm oil over medium-high warmth up until hot. Throw eggplant with flour and also fry until golden. Transfer to a paper towel-lined plate.
2. Include onion to skillet along with garlic clove. Include tomatoes, season with Salt and pepper, as well as cook for concerning 10 minutes; after that pass mixture through a food mill. Include eggplant to tomato Sauce
3. Bring a pot of well-salted water to a boil. Cook rigatoni up until al dente, drain, and also pour it into a large dish. Add Sauce, mix, and then include basil. Transfer to bowls, spray with ricotta salata, and also serve.

Pasta with Cannellini Beans

Prep Time: 10 min
Cook Time: 25 min
Servings: 4

INGREDIENTS

- 1 small onion, chopped
- 2 garlic cloves, minced
- 2 tablespoons olive oil
- 1 teaspoon salt
- 2 cups canned crushed tomatoes
- 1 cup water
- 1½ cups elbow-shaped pasta
- 2 (16-ounce) cans cannellini beans, rinsed and drained

DIRECTIONS

1. In a large sauté pan over low heat, combine the onion, garlic, oil, and salt, and simmer for 1 to 2 minutes, paying close attention that the garlic does not burn. Add the tomatoes and water, and simmer over low to medium heat for 18 minutes.
2. In the meantime, cook the pasta in salted boiling water as directed on the package.
3. When the sauce is cooked, add the beans. Over low heat, cook the beans and sauce for 5 minutes, gently folding the beans into the sauce.
4. Add the cooked pasta, and gently fold in all the ingredients to incorporate. Serve hot.

Maccheroni with Cauliflower

Prep Time: 24 min
Cook Time: 1 hour
Servings: 4

INGREDIENTS

- 1 large head cauliflower, core and cut into
- 1-1/2" pieces
- 10 cloves of garlic, peeled
- 1-28 oz. can crushed San Marzano Tomatoes
- 1 medium onion, minced
- ½ teaspoon crushed red pepper flakes
- ¼ cup olive oil, salt and pepper to taste

OPTIONAL BREADCRUMB TOPPING

- 6 tablespoons Olive Oil
- 2 cloves Garlic, peeled and minced fine
- ½ plain Breadcrumbs

DIRECTIONS

1. Place half the oil in a large pot with the minced onions. Sauté for three minutes. Add five cloves of garlic that have been thinly sliced. Sauté for 3 minutes over low heat. Add Red Pepper, sauté for 2 minutes.
2. Add tomatoes and simmer over low heat for 25 minutes.
3. While tomato sauce is simmering, place remainder of olive oil in a large frying pan and sauté the cauliflower over medium heat for 12-15 minutes until it is slightly browned.
4. Add remaining Five whole Garlic cloves with the Cauliflower, and sauté for about 5 minutes. Add salt and pepper to taste. Add cauliflower to tomato sauce and cook for 10 minutes.
5. You can use almost any pasta for this sauce, although short pasta such as Rigatoni, Ditalini, Orecchietti, or Cavatappi work best.
6. Cook the pasta according to directions on package. Drain the pasta in a colander. Put pasta back in the pot it cooked in, add ¾ of the sauce over pasta and mix.
7. To serve, plate the pasta, topping each plate with some additional Cauliflower Sauce. Pass the grated Pecorino Romano or Parmigiano Reggiano Cheese.
8. Note: The Breadcrumb topping is optional if you'd like to use it. The breadcrumb topping is quite tradition in Sicilian Pasta dishes as it came about as a substitute for grated cheese, which was too expensive for many Sicilians in years past, so they used these breadcrumbs. Try it sometimes, it's makes for a nice alternative.

Lentil Bolognese

Prep Time: 8 min
Cook Time: 25 min
Servings: 4

INGREDIENTS

- 1 small white onion, diced
- 3 garlic cloves, minced
- 1 large zucchini, diced small
- 8 oz. (226 g) (1 cup/235 ml) button mushrooms, diced
- 1 teaspoon (5 ml) basil
- 1 teaspoon (5 ml) salt
- ½ teaspoon (2.5 ml) black pepper
- 1 14 oz. (~400 g or similar size) (1 2/3cups/400 ml) can fire-roasted diced tomatoes
- 3 cups (700 ml) pasta sauce
- 1 cup (235 ml) brown lentils, rinsed
- 2 cups (470 ml) water
- 1 lb. (0.5 kg) (4½ cups/1060 ml) linguine pasta

DIRECTIONS

1. Place the olive oil into a saucepot and heat it over medium-high heat.
2. Stir in the onion, garlic, zucchini, button mushrooms, basil, salt, and pepper and cook for 3-5 minutes until the onions become translucent.
3. Stir in the tomatoes, pasta sauce, lentils, and water, and bring the Bolognese to a boil.
4. Decrease the flame to medium-low and cook the Bolognese for 20-25 minutes, periodically stirring until the lentils are tender.
5. Cook the linguini pasta according to the manufacturer's instructions, drain it, then divide the pasta between 4 bowls, then top with the lentil Bolognese sauce.
6. Serve and enjoy!

Pasta

Pasta with Garlic and Oil

Prep Time 2 min | **Cook Time** 10 min | **Servings** 4

INGREDIENTS
- 16 ounces spaghetti
- Salt
- ¼ cup extra-virgin olive oil
- Red pepper flakes
- 4 large garlic cloves, minced
- 1 tablespoon chopped fresh parsley
- ¼ cup grated Pecorino Romano cheese

DIRECTIONS
1. Cook the spaghetti in salted boiling water per the package instructions.
2. When the spaghetti is nearly cooked, in a medium sauté pan over low heat, heat the oil. Add red pepper flakes to taste and the garlic, and cook until the garlic turns color, paying close attention that it does not burn.
3. Drain the pasta, reserving some of the liquid. Add the spaghetti to the pan and toss well to coat. Add a few tablespoons of the pasta water and continue tossing until the water is evaporated.
4. Remove from the heat and add the parsley and cheese. Serve hot.

Green Tomato Pasta

Prep Time 15 min | **Cook Time** 30 min | **Servings** 4

INGREDIENTS
- 4 cups spaghetti
- 4 large green tomatoes, thinly sliced (1/8-inch thick)
- Salt and pepper, to taste
- 1 cup flour
- Vegetable oil, for frying
- 2 garlic cloves, minced
- 1/4 cup parmesan cheese, grated

DIRECTIONS
1. Prepare spaghetti according to package directions; drain well and set aside.
2. Season tomatoes with salt and pepper. Coat with flour and fry in hot oil with garlic until golden brown. Do not overcook. Place fried tomato slices on top of hot, cooked pasta. Top with parmesan cheese and serve immediately.

Pasta with Bread Crumbs

Prep Time 5 min | **Cook Time** 12 min | **Servings** 4

INGREDIENTS
- ¾ pound fusilli pasta (or other pasta of choice)
- 3 tablespoons extra-virgin olive oil, plus more for drizzling
- 1 cup fresh bread crumbs (see tip)
- 5 or 6 anchovies (optional)
- 2 tablespoons chopped fresh parsley
- ½ cup grated Pecorino Romano cheese (or other grated cheese)

1. Cook the pasta for 2 minutes less than instructed on the package. Drain, reserving ¼ cup of the pasta water. Meanwhile, in a medium sauté pan over medium-high heat, heat the oil. Add the bread crumbs and toast for several minutes. Add the anchovies (if using), and cook with the crumbs until the anchovies break down and dissolve completely. Add the pasta to the bread crumbs and toast for several additional minutes, mixing all the ingredients. If wetter pasta is desired, add a few tablespoons of the pasta water.
2. Add the parsley and cheese and remove from the heat. Top with an additional drizzle of oil. Serve immediately.

Pistachio Pasta

Prep Time: 10 min
Cook Time: 15 min
Servings: 4

INGREDIENTS

- 1 (8 oz.) box penne pasta, cooked, drained
- 2 tablespoons butter
- 1 large yellow onion, thinly sliced
- 1/2 cup green bell pepper, diced
- 1/2 cup red bell pepper, diced
- 2 tablespoons garlic, minced
- 1/4 lb. prosciutto, diced
- 1 cup pistachios, coarsely chopped
- 1 (2.25) can sliced olives
- 1 1/2 teaspoons dried rosemary crumbled
- 1/2 cup extra-virgin olive oil
- 4 oz. blue cheese, crumbled

DIRECTIONS

1. Cook pasta according to package directions; drain and set aside.
2. Melt butter. In a large skillet, sauté onion until tender. Add peppers, garlic, prosciutto, pistachios, olives, rosemary and olive oil to skillet. Continue cooking, stirring until hot. Add crumbled blue cheese. Toss with pasta and serve

Norcina Style Pasta

Prep Time: 15 min
Cook Time: 20 min
Servings: 6

INGREDIENTS

- 3 tablespoons olive oil
- 2 garlic cloves, minced
- 6 pork sausages, casings removed
- ½ cup dry white wine
- ¾ cup heavy cream
- ¾ pound pasta, such as rigatoni, ziti, or penne
- Salt
- ¼ cup grated Parmesan cheese

DIRECTIONS

1. In a large sauté pan over medium heat, combine the oil, garlic, and sausage. Use a wooden spoon to crumble the sausage until it resembles ground meat. Add the wine and cook for about 10 minutes.
2. Add the cream, reduce the heat to low, and cook for an additional 5 minutes. Meanwhile, cook the pasta in salted boiling water for 2 minutes less than directed on the package. Drain, reserving ¼ cup of the pasta water.
3. Add the pasta to the sauce, stirring well to coat the pasta. Continue cooking until the pasta is fully cooked and all the flavors are well incorporated. Add a few tablespoons of the pasta water if a thinner sauce is desired.
4. Remove from the heat and add the cheese, stirring well to incorporate. Serve immediately.

Pasta

Eggplant Pasta

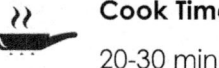

Prep Time: 30 min
Cook Time: 20-30 min
Servings: 6

INGREDIENTS

- 2 small eggplants, chopped into 1/2-inch cubes (about 5 to 6 cups)
- 1 large onion, chopped
- 1/4 cup extra-virgin olive oil, divided
- 4 stalks celery, sliced
- 2 large green bell peppers, chopped
- 2 to 4 cloves garlic, minced
- 1 (28 oz.) can diced tomatoes, with juice
- 3 to 4 tablespoons red wine vinegar
- 1/2 teaspoon salt
- Pepper, to taste
- 8 oz. rotelle pasta, cooked
- 1/4 cup Parmesan cheese, grated

DIRECTIONS

1. Soak eggplant in salted water for 15 minutes; drain. Meanwhile, sauté onion in 2 tablespoons olive oil. Add celery; sauté until bright green. Add peppers and garlic; sauté 2 to 3 minutes. Add tomatoes with their liquid, vinegar and salt. Remove from pan and set aside.
2. Add remaining oil to pan and sauté eggplant until tender. Return tomato mixture to pan and heat through. Serve over cooked rotelle and garnish with cheese.

Baked Stuffed Shells

Prep Time: 25 min
Cook Time: 1 h and 10 min
Servings: 6

INGREDIENTS

- ¼ cup extra-virgin olive oil
- 1/3 cup chopped fresh Italian parsley
- ½ teaspoon crushed red pepper flakes
- 1 big egg
- 1 cup freshly grated Grana Padano
- 1 pound fresh mozzarella cheese
- 1 pound jumbo pasta shells
- 10 fresh basil leaves
- 1½ pounds fresh ricotta or packaged whole milk ricotta, drained overnight
- 6 garlic cloves, crushed and peeled
- Freshly ground black pepper to taste
- Kosher salt
- One 35-ounce can peeled Italian plum tomatoes, if possible San Marzano, crushed using your hands

DIRECTIONS

1. Preheat your oven to 425 degrees. Bring a big pot of salted water to its boiling point for the pasta. Heat the olive oil in a big frying pan on moderate heat. Spread the garlic over the oil, and cook, shaking the pan, until a golden-brown colour is achieved, approximately two minutes. Pour the tomatoes into the frying pan, slosh out the can with 1 cup water, and put in that. Put in the crushed red pepper, and sprinkle lightly with salt. Bring the sauce to a quick boil, then regulate the heat to simmering. Cook until the sauce is a little thickened, approximately half an hour. Mix the basil into the sauce a few minutes before it is done.
2. Mix the shells into the salted boiling water, and cook, stirring once in a while, until a little firmer than firm to the bite, approximately seven minutes. Fish the shells out of the water using a spider, and plunge into a big bowl of ice water. Allow to cool, then drain.
3. Thinly slice half the mozzarella, and chop the rest of the half into ¼-inch cubes. Turn the drained ricotta into a mixing bowl, and mix in the mozzarella cubes, grated cheese, and parsley. Sprinkle salt and pepper to taste. Beat the egg well, and stir it into the ricotta mixture.
4. Take the garlic and line the bottom of a 10-by-fifteen-inch baking dish with approximately ¾ cup of the tomato sauce. Spoon about 2 tablespoons of the ricotta mixture into each shell—the shell must be filled to capacity, but not overstuffed. Nestle the shells next to each other in the baking dish as you fill them, spooning the rest of the sauce over the shells, coating each one. Position the slices of mozzarella in a uniform layer over the shells. Bake until the mozzarella is browned and bubbling, approximately twenty-five minutes. Take out of the oven, and allow it to stand five minutes before you serve.

Tofu Spinach Lasagna

Prep Time: 45 min
Cook Time: 30 min
Servings: 12

INGREDIENTS

- 9 lasagna noodles
- 1 medium onion, chopped
- 3 garlic cloves, minced
- 1 tablespoon olive oil
- 2 cups sliced fresh mushrooms
- 1 package (14 ounces) firm tofu
- 1 carton (15 ounces) part-skim ricotta cheese
- 1/2 cup minced fresh parsley
- 1 teaspoon salt, divided
- 2 packages (10 ounces each) frozen chopped spinach, thawed and squeezed dry
- 1-3/4 cups marinara or meatless spaghetti sauce
- 1 cup shredded part-skim mozzarella cheese
- 1/3 cup shredded Parmesan cheese

DIRECTIONS

1. Follow the instructions at the back of the package in cooking the noodles. For the meantime, cook garlic and onion with oil on a large nonstick pan for about 60 seconds. Mix in mushrooms and cook until it's soft. Put aside.
2. Save 2 tbsp. of liquid from the tofu then discard the rest. On a covered food processor, blend the saved liquid and the tofu. Put in ricotta cheese. Put the cover back and blend again for 60-120 seconds until smooth. Pour it onto a large bowl and add half teaspoon of salt, mushroom mixture and parsley. Mix in the remaining salt and spinach then let it rest.
3. Drain the cooked noodles. Grease a 13x9-inch baking pan with cooking spray. Pour half of the marinara sauce in it and arrange three noodles, 1/2 of the tofu mixture, and 1/2 of the spinach mixture in layer. Do the layers of the noodles, tofu mixture, and spinach mixture again. Place the remaining noodles and marinara sauce on top. Put cheese over.
4. Let it bake, unsealed, for 30-35 minutes at 350°F. Bake until the cheese has melted and until heated through. Leave for ten minutes before cutting and serving.

NUTRITION: Calories: 227 Calories | Fiber: 3g | Carbs: 25g | Protein: 15g protein | Fat: 8g fat | Sodium: 429mg sodium

Italian Lasagna

Prep Time: 20 min
Cook Time: 5.5-7.5 min
Servings: 15

INGREDIENTS

- 9 thick slices bacon, diced
- 1 onion, chopped
- 1 teaspoon fennel seed
- 1 teaspoon dried oregano
- 1 ½ teaspoons Italian seasoning
- 2 (28 ounce) cans tomato sauce
- 2 pounds Italian sausage
- 1 (16 ounce) package lasagna noodles
- 2 pints part-skim ricotta cheese
- 2 large eggs
- 2 teaspoons chopped fresh parsley
- 1 teaspoon dried oregano
- 1/3 cup milk
- 8 slices provolone cheese
- 6 cups shredded mozzarella cheese

DIRECTIONS

1. Brown the bacon and onion in a large skillet over medium heat. Toss together fennel seed, 1 teaspoon oregano, Italian spice, and tomato sauce. Cook for 4 to 6 hours on low, or until the sauce has thickened.
2. In a large skillet, brown the sausage links. Using paper towels, absorb any excess liquid. Cut each piece into 1 inch sections.
3. Layer 1 cup of sauce on the bottom of a 9 x 13 inch pan. 1/3 uncooked lasagna noodles, 1/2 ricotta cheese mixture, 1/2 sausage bits, 1/3 mozzarella, and 1/2 provolone cheese should be layered on top. 1/3 of the sauce should be on top. Layers should be repeated. Add the remaining 1/3 of the noodles on top. Spread the remaining sauce on top and top with the remaining 1/3 of the mozzarella cheese.
4. Preheat oven to 350°F (175°C) and bake for 1 1/2 hours

NUTRITION: Calories 754.8 Cal | Protein 40.2g | Carbohydrates 34.4g Fat 51g | Cholesterol 156.1mg | Sodium 1701.9

Pasta

Italian Savory Bread Pasta

Prep Time 10 min **Cook Time** 20 min **Servings** 8

INGREDIENTS

- 6 cup chicken stock
- 8 oz pasta noodles
- 2 tablespoon tomato sauce
- 1 teaspoon paprika
- 1 tablespoon butter
- 1 teaspoon Italian seasoning
- ½ teaspoon chili flakes
- 1 teaspoon minced garlic
- 1 cup breadcrumbs
- ¼ teaspoon dried dill

DIRECTIONS

1. Pour the chicken stock into the saucepan and preheat it.
2. Add the pasta noodles and cook them according to the directions of the manufacturer.
3. Meanwhile, combine the breadcrumbs with the dried dill and paprika.
4. Add chili flakes and stir the breadcrumbs mixture.
5. When the pasta noodles are cooked – strain them in the colander and add butter.
6. Combine the tomato sauce with the Italian seasoning, minced garlic, and mix the mixture up.
7. Transfer the pasta noodles in the big bowl and sprinkle with the tomato sauce mixture and stir it.
8. Then sprinkle the cooked dish with the bread crumbs and stir it gently.
9. Transfer the prepared dish to the serving plates.

NUTRITION: Calories 133 Cal | Fat 4g | Fiber 2 g | Carbohydrates 17.88 g | Protein 6g

---

Italian Shrimp Caprese Pasta

Prep Time 25 min **Cook Time** 25 min **Servings** 4

INGREDIENTS

- 8 ounces dried linguine
- 1 lb. medium uncooked shrimp, deveined
- 1 cup grape tomatoes, cut in halves
- 1 cup fresh mozzarella, cubed
- 4 tbsp chopped fresh basil leaves
- 4 tbsp shredded Parmesan cheese
- 2 squares of Italian Herb Saute Express

DIRECTIONS

1. Drain pasta after cooking according to package directions.
2. In a 12-inch nonstick skillet, melt Saute Express® squares over medium-low heat until bubbles form. Toss in the shrimp.
3. Cook until the shrimp are pink, for about 5 to 7 minutes. Stir in the pasta, tomatoes, mozzarella, and basil until thoroughly coated and cooked. Parmesan cheese should be sprinkled on top.

NUTRITION: Calories 471 Cal | Protein 35.1g | Carbohydrates 44.6g Fat 17.4g | Sodium 729.3mg

Fusilli with Chicken RAGÙ

Prep Time: 20 min | **Cook Time:** 45 min | **Servings:** 6

INGREDIENTS

- ¼ cup chopped fresh Italian parsley
- ¼ cup extra-virgin olive oil, plus more for drizzling
- ¼ teaspoon crushed red pepper flakes
- ½ cup freshly grated Grana Padano
- ½ cup white wine
- 1 fresh bay leaf
- 1 pound boneless, skinless chicken thighs, trimmed of fat and sinew, cut into ½-inch chunks
- 1 pound fusilli
- 1 teaspoon kosher salt, plus more for the pot
- 1½ cups frozen peas
- 2 celery stalks, diced
- 2 cups Chicken Stock
- 3 medium artichokes, cleaned, halved, and cut
- 3 medium leeks, white and light green parts, halved, washed, and thinly cut
- Grated zest of 1 lemon

DIRECTIONS

1. Bring a big pot of salted water to its boiling point for the pasta. Heat a medium Dutch oven on moderate to high heat. Put in the olive oil. When the oil is hot, put in the leeks, artichokes, and celery. Flavor it with ½ teaspoon salt and the red pepper flakes. Toss to coat the vegetables in the oil, and cook until they start to wilt, approximately five minutes.
2. Push the vegetables to the side of the pan, and put in the chicken in the empty space. Season the chicken with the rest of the ½ teaspoon salt. Toss the chicken in the empty space until it is no longer raw on the outside, then mix into the vegetables. Put in the wine, and cook quickly until reduced by half, approximately two minutes. Put in the chicken stock and bay leaf, and bring to a simmer. Partly cover, and simmer until the chicken and vegetables are super soft, approximately twenty minutes.
3. Remove the cover, put in the peas, and simmer, uncovered, to reduce and concentrate the sauce while you cook the pasta. Remove bay leaf and discard. Put in the pasta to the boiling water. When the pasta is firm to the bite, remove using a spider and move directly to the simmering sauce. Put in the parsley, lemon zest, and a sprinkle of olive oil. Toss to coat the pasta in the sauce, putting in a little pasta water if it appears dry. Take the frying pan from the heat, drizzle with the grated cheese, toss, before you serve.

Pepperoni Pasta

Prep Time: 25 min | **Cook Time:** 55 min | **Servings:** 6-8

INGREDIENTS

- 1 lb. ground beef
- 1 medium onion, chopped
- 1 medium green pepper, chopped
- 1 garlic clove, minced
- 3-1/2 cups spaghetti sauce
- 1 can (4 oz.) mushroom stems and pieces, drained
- 1 package (3-1/2 oz.) sliced pepperoni
- 8 oz. uncooked spiral pasta, wagon wheel pasta or pastas of your choice
- 1 cup shredded part-skim mozzarella cheese
- 1 cup shredded provolone cheese
- Grated Parmesan cheese

DIRECTIONS

1. On medium heat, cook green pepper, onion, and beef in a big skillet until the meat is not pink anymore. Put in garlic then cook for another minute; drain. Put in pepperoni, mushrooms, and spaghetti sauce.
2. Put 1/2 of the pasta and meat mixture in a layer in a greased 13-in by 9-in baking dish. Top with half cup each of provolone and mozzarella cheeses. Repeat the layers then scatter with Parmesan cheese.
3. Bake for 30-35 mins in a 400 degrees F oven without a cover or until thoroughly heated. Let it sit for 15 mins Serve.

NUTRITION: Calories: 372 Calories | Total CarbS: 22 g | Cholesterol: 61 mg | Total Fat: 21 g | Fiber: 3 g | Protein: 23 g Sodium: 992 mg |

Pasta

Baked Elbows with Pork RAGÙ

Prep Time: 25 min
Cook Time: 1 hour 25 min approx
Servings: 6

INGREDIENTS

- ¼ cup extra-virgin olive oil
- ½ teaspoon crushed red pepper flakes
- ¾ cup freshly grated Grana Padano
- 1 celery stalk, cut into chunks
- 1 cup dry white wine
- 1 medium carrot, peeled and slice into chunks
- 1 medium onion, cut into chunks
- 1 pound elbow macaroni
- 1 tablespoon unsalted butter, softened
- 1½ pounds boneless pork shoulder, trimmed of most of the fat and sinews, cut into 1-inch chunks
- 2 cups grated low-moisture mozzarella
- 2 garlic cloves, crushed and peeled
- 2 medium zucchini, cut into ¼-inch-thick rounds
- 2 tablespoons fine dried bread crumbs
- 2 teaspoons kosher salt, plus more for the pot
- One 28-ounce can Italian plum tomatoes, if possible San Marzano, crushed using your hands

DIRECTIONS

1. Preheat your oven to 375 degrees. Bring a big pot of salted water to its boiling point for the pasta. Butter a nine by thirteen-inch baking dish. Drizzle with the bread crumbs, and tap to coat the interior of the dish, tapping out the surplus. Run the pork shoulder through the coarse holes of a meat grinder. (You can also use pre-ground pork or sausage, but the crudely ground texture is preferred.)
2. Use a food processor to mix the onion, carrot, celery, and garlic. Process to make a smooth pestata. To a big Dutch oven on moderate to high heat, put in the olive oil. When the oil is hot, put in the pestata, and cook until it dries out and is light golden, approximately five minutes. Put in the ground pork, and flavor with the salt and crushed red pepper. Lower the heat to moderate, and cook until the pork releases its juices, approximately seven minutes. Raise the heat to get the juices boiling, and cook until they're reduced away and the pork is browned, approximately five minutes. Put in the white wine, and cook until reduced by half, approximately two minutes. Put in the tomatoes, slosh out the can with 1 cup pasta water, and put in that, too. Heat to a simmer, and cook until the pork is soft, approximately half an hour.
3. Put in the zucchini, and cook until it is soft and the sauce is thick, approximately twenty minutes more.
4. When the zucchini is almost done, cook the elbows in the boiling water until just firm to the bite (they will cook more as they bake). Drain, saving for later 1 cup pasta water. In a moderate-sized bowl, toss the mozzarella and grated Grana Padano together.
5. When the sauce is ready, put in the elbows and toss to coat the pasta in the sauce, putting in a splash of pasta water if it appears dry. Take the pot from the heat, and fold in half of the cheese mixture. Spread the pasta in the readied pan, and drizzle with the rest of the cheese mixture. Bake until the sauce is bubbly and the top is brown and crusty, approximately twenty-five minutes. Allow it to sit five minutes before you serve.

No-bake Mushroom Lasagna

Prep Time: 20 min
Cook Time: 30 min
Servings: 6

INGREDIENTS

- 2 lasagna noodles
- 1/4 cup sliced fresh mushrooms
- 2 tbsps. chopped onion
- 1 tsp. canola oil
- 1/2 cup spaghetti sauce
- 1/4 cup chopped tomato
- 1/8 tsp. dried basil
- Dash pepper
- 1/4 cup shredded part-skim mozzarella cheese
- 2 tsps. shredded Parmesan cheese

DIRECTIONS

1. Prepare the lasagna noodles following the package instructions. Sauté onions and mushroom in a small pan until tender. Put in pepper, spaghetti sauce, basil, and tomato; boil. Lower heat and let it simmer, covered, for 10 mins; mix from time to time. On low heat, cook in mozzarella cheese until it melts
2. Cut drained noodles into thirds. Spread 2 tbsps. sauce on a plate and top with 2 noodle pieces. Repeat the process for another two times. Add the leftover sauce and top with Parmesan cheese.

NUTRITION: Calories: 430 Calories | Total CarbS: 55 g | Cholesterol: 22 mg Total Fat: 15 g | Fiber: 5 g | Protein: 19 g | Sodium: 814 mg

Braised Octopus with Spaghetti

Prep Time: 20 min
Cook Time: 2 hour 3/4
Servings: 6

INGREDIENTS

- ¼ teaspoon kosher salt, plus more for the pot
- ½ cup extra-virgin olive oil
- 1 cup Gaeta or other black brine-cured olives, pitted
- 1 pound spaghetti
- 2 big onions, thinly cut (approximately four cups)
- 2 cleaned octopuses (about 2½ pounds total)
- 2 tablespoons chopped fresh Italian parsley

DIRECTIONS

1. Heat 6 tablespoons of the olive oil in a moderate-sized (4-to-6-quart) deep cooking pan or Dutch oven using low heat. Spread the onion slices over the bottom of the pan, and lay the octopuses on top. Spread the olives over the octopuses, cover the pan, and allow the octopuses to heat slowly, releasing their liquid, and beginning to cook in it.

2. After around sixty minutes, uncover the pan and check to see that there is plenty of octopus liquid in the pan. If it appears dry, put in 1 cup of water at a time. This recipe should yield 2 cups of sauce when the octopuses are done. Carry on the covered slow cooking for one more hour, until the octopuses are super soft. Begin testing for doneness after 1¾ hours: stick the tines of a fork in the thickest part of each octopus; when the fork slides out easily, the meat is done.

3. Take the octopuses from the pot, and allow them to cool a little. To make a meaty octopus sauce: cut both octopuses into ¾-inch chunks, skin and all (or you can leave the octopuses whole for serving). Measure the liquid rest of the in the deep cooking pan. Again, you should have about 2 cups total. If the volume is greater, return the juices to the deep cooking pan and boil to reduce them. Place the cut octopus meat and the juices in the frying pan for dressing the pasta.

4. In the meantime, bring a big pot of salted water to its boiling point for the pasta. Put in the spaghetti. As the spaghetti cooks, bring the octopus meat and sauce in the frying pan to a rapid simmer; taste, and put in ¼ teaspoon salt if required (octopus is naturally salty). Mix in the parsley. Take the spaghetti using tongs and move directly to the sauce. Toss to coat the pasta with the sauce, putting in a splash of pasta water if it appears dry. Remove the heat, sprinkle over the rest of the 2 tablespoons olive oil, and toss once more. Heap the spaghetti into warm bowls, ensuring each portion gets plenty of octopus pieces, and serve instantly.

Pasta

Spinach Tortelloni

Prep Time 15 min **Cook Time** 20 min **Servings** 6

- Pasta
- ½ teaspoon extra-virgin olive oil
- ½ teaspoon kosher salt
- 4 cups all-purpose flour, plus more as required
- 6 big eggs
- Filling
- ½ cup freshly grated Grana Padano
- 1 big egg, whisked
- 1 cup frozen spinach, thawed
- 1 pound fresh ricotta
- 8 ounces ricotta salata, grated
- Freshly ground black pepper
- Sauce
- ½ cup freshly grated Grana Padano
- 1½ cups heavy cream
- 1½ sticks unsalted butter
- Freshly ground black pepper
- Kosher salt

1. To make the pasta using your hands: Make a mound of 3½ cups of the flour on a countertop or big wooden board, and form a well in the middle. In a spouted measuring cup, combine the eggs, olive oil, and salt. Cautiously pour the mixture into the well, ensuring it doesn't break through the sides. Use a fork to flick flour from the inside edges of the well into the egg mixture, mixing as you go. Stir in sufficient flour to make a sticky dough; then, use a bench scraper to mix the remaining flour into the mixture. Put in up to ½ cup of the rest of the flour to make a dough that will form a ball without clinging to your hands. (It's okay if you don't use all of the flour.) Knead until smooth and satiny, flouring your hands as you go to keep the dough from adhering. Cover the dough with plastic wrap, and allow it to rest at room temperature for an hour.

2. To make dough in the food processor: Pulse 3½ cups of the flour and the salt together. Combine the eggs and olive oil together in a spouted measuring cup, and pour into the flour while the machine runs. Process until the dough forms a tender ball on the blade, putting in up to ½ cup of the rest of the flour if required. Run the dough in the processor approximately twenty to half a minute to knead it; it must be smooth and glossy but still flexible. Turn the dough onto a mildly floured work surface, and knead just a few times, to bring it together. Cover it using plastic wrap and allow it to rest 1 hour at room temperature.

3. For the filling: Place the thawed spinach in a kitchen towel, and squeeze out as much liquid as you can. Finely cut the spinach, and put it in a big bowl. Put in the ricotta, ricotta salata, Grana Padano, egg, and some pepper, and mix thoroughly.

4. Chop the dough into four equivalent portions. Keep the other pieces covered as you start to roll one. Prepare two baking sheets. Push the dough into a rectangle, and roll through the pasta machine; fold in half, and roll through once more. Fold the dough in three like a letter and roll through again, with the folded ends at the side. Repeat this folding and rolling multiple times, every time lowering the setting on the machine until you reach the second-last setting, to toughen and lengthen the dough. Repeat this step with the rest of the three pieces of dough, keeping the others floured and covered with kitchen towels while you work.

5. Switch to the third setting on the pasta machine, and roll each piece through a couple of times, with the short end going in first. Reset pasta machine to the fifth setting, and roll the pieces through. They will get much longer this time, so cut each piece in half crosswise. You should have eight long pieces now, all around the width of the machine. Roll each piece once through the second-last setting.

6. Coat rolled sheets of dough between clean kitchen towels. Work with one sheet of rolled dough at a time. Fill a small bowl with water. Use a three-inch round cutter to cut as many discs as you can from one strip of dough, keeping the other strips covered while you work. Spoon a loaded teaspoon of filling in each round. Wet the edges with a finger dipped in water, and fold over, making a half-moon; press firmly to secure the edges and press out surplus air. Arrange each piece around your index finger, with the filled part on the fingernail. Bring the two edges to meet on the front of your finger, and press the ends together, making a ring. Slide it off your finger onto a floured sheet pan. Repeat with the rest of the dough circles, keeping all the dough covered while you work.

7. Bring a big pot of salted water to its boiling point for the pasta. For the sauce: In a big frying pan on moderate to high heat, melt the butter. When the butter is melted, pour in the cream and adjust the heat so the sauce is simmering quickly. Simmer until the sauce is reduced by approximately one-third, approximately six to seven minutes.

8. When the sauce is almost done, cook the tortelloni. Put in them to the boiling water and cook until firm to the bite, approximately two to three minutes from the time they float. Take the tortelloni using a spider, and put in directly to the simmering sauce. Toss gently to coat the pasta with the sauce, and sprinkle with salt and pepper, putting in a little pasta water if it appears dry, or reducing it using high heat for one minute if it's too soupy. Take the frying pan from the heat. Drizzle with the grated cheese, toss, and serve instantly.

Special Italian Easter Pizza

Prep Time 40 min **Cook Time** 50 min **Servings** 10

INGREDIENTS

- ½ pound bulk Italian sausage
- 2 teaspoons olive oil
- 1 pound loaf frozen bread dough, thawed
- ½ pound sliced mozzarella cheese
- ½ pound sliced ham, cooked
- ½ pound sliced provolone cheese
- ½ pound sliced salami
- ½ pound sliced pepperoni
- 1 container (16 ounce) ricotta cheese
- ½ cup grated Parmesan cheese
- 8 large eggs, beaten
- 1 egg
- 1 teaspoon water
- (springform pan needed)

DIRECTIONS

1. Cook and stir Italian sausage in a pan over medium heat until fully browned, 5 to 8 minutes, breaking the sausage into chunks as it cooks.
2. Remove the sausage from the pan. Drain any extra fat.
3. Preheat the oven to 350 deg. Fahrenheit (175 degrees C).
4. Olive oil the bottom and sides of a 10-inch springform pan.
5. Remove the one third portion of the dough from the loaf and lay it aside under a damp cloth. Roll out the remaining the dough into a 14-inch circle.
6. Roll out the dough and line the pan, allowing 2 inches of dough to hang over the edge all around.
7. In the pie crust, layer half of the cooked Italian sausage, half of the mozzarella cheese, half of the ham, half of the provolone cheese, half of the salami, and half of the pepperoni.
8. Spoon Half of the ricotta cheese and put over the layers of meat and cheeses.
9. Sprinkle half the Parmesan cheese over the ricotta.
10. Layer the remaining meats, sliced cheeses, ricotta cheese, and then Parmesan cheese on top of half of the 8 beaten eggs.
11. Over the last layer of Parmesan cheese, pour the remaining beaten eggs.
12. Roll out the remaining piece of bread dough into a 12 inch circle and place it on top of the pie to . This will be used top crust of pie.
13. To seal in the filling, roll and pinch the bottom crust excess over the top crust. In a tiny bowl, whisk together water and one egg; brush the egg wash over the top of the pie.
14. In a preheated oven, bake the pie for 50 to 60 minutes, until the filling is set and the crust is golden brown and. A toothpick inserted in the center of the crust should come out clean.
15. Allow for at least 25 minutes of cooling time in the pan before releasing the spring and removing the pie. Cut into wedges before serving.

Nutrition: Calories 707.3 Cal | Protein 45.4g | Carbs 28.1g | Fat 44.6g | Cholesterol 283.5mg | Sodium 2090.3mg

Pasta

Rice

Prep Time 15 min | **Cook Time** 18 min | **Servings** 4

INGREDIENTS
- 2 cups Arborio rice
- 6 fresh basil leaves, minced
- 4 tablespoons freshly grated Pecorino Romano cheese
- 1/2 tablespoons olive oil
- Salt to taste
- 2 medium tomatoes, cut into thin wedges, for garnish
- Fresh parsley sprigs, for garnish

DIRECTIONS
1. Bring 4 quarts lightly salted water to a boil in a large saucepan. Add the rice and cook, checking for doneness after approximately 18 minutes. Rice should be al dente, or firm to the bite; do not overcook. When the rice is done, remove from the heat, pour into a colander, and toss gently to remove excess water.
2. Place the hot rice in a large mixing bowl and add the basil and cheese. Stir gently to combine, then add the olive oil and toss thoroughly. Season with salt.
3. Spoon the hot rice mixture into a 2-quart mold and press gently to set. Immediately unmold the rice onto a large serving platter. Garnish with tomato wedges and parsley sprigs.

Classic Paella Simple

Prep Time 10 min | **Cook Time** 25 min | **Servings** 4

INGREDIENTS
- 10 ounces risotto rice
- 12 ounces mixed shrimp and sea scallops, cooked and frozen
- 14 ounces canned tomatoes, chopped
- 1-quart chicken stock
- Juice of ½ lemon
- ½ lemon cut into wedges
- A handful parsley, chopped
- Salt and black pepper to the taste
- 1 yellow onion, chopped
- 1 teaspoon smoked paprika
- 1 teaspoon thyme, dried
- 3 tablespoons sherry
- 1 tablespoon extra-virgin olive oil

DIRECTIONS
1. Heat up a pan with the oil over medium high heat, add onion, stir and cook for 5 minutes.
2. Add thyme, rice and paprika, stir and cook for 1 minute.
3. Add sherry, stir and cook for 1 minute more.
4. Add tomatoes and stock and cook for 15 minutes stirring from time to time.
5. Add salt and pepper to the taste, seafood mix and lemon juice, stir and cook for 5 minutes more.
6. Sprinkle parsley, stir, divide into bowls and serve with lemon wedges on the side.

Nutrition: Calories 430 Cal | Fat 4g | Fiber 2g | Carbohydrates 33g | Protein 25g

Rice Balls

Prep Time

Cook Time

Servings — 24 rice balls

INGREDIENTS

- ½ teaspoon kosher salt, plus more for seasoning
- 1 cup all-purpose flour
- 1 cup dry white wine
- 1 cup finely diced ham or prosciutto (about 3 ounces)
- 1 cup freshly grated Grana Padano
- 1 cup frozen peas, thawed
- 1 medium onion, chopped
- 10 basil leaves, chopped
- 2 big eggs
- 2 cups Arborio rice
- 2 cups fine dried bread crumbs
- 3 tablespoons extra-virgin olive oil
- 4 ounces fresh mozzarella, cut into 24 cubes
- 5 cups Chicken Stock
- Vegetable oil, for frying

DIRECTIONS

1. In a small pot, warm chicken stock over low heat. In a moderate-sized deep cooking pan, heat the olive oil. When the oil is hot, put in the onion and cook until it starts to soften, approximately three to four minutes. Put in the ham or prosciutto, and cook a few minutes, until it starts to render its fat. Put in the rice, and cook to coat it in the oil and fat. Pour in the wine, bring to a simmer, and cook until the wine is almost reduced away. Put in 3 cups of the hot chicken stock and the salt. Cover, and simmer until the chicken stock is absorbed by the rice, approximately seven to eight minutes. Put in the rest of the 2 cups stock, and cover once more. Cook until rice is al dente, approximately six to seven minutes more. Uncover; if any liquid remains, increase heat and cook until all of the liquid is absorbed, one more minute or two. Mix in peas, and spread rice on a rimmed sheet pan to cool.
2. Once the rice cools down, put in a container and stir in grated cheese and chopped basil. Scoop out about 1/3 cup rice, and place a cube of mozzarella in the center, making a firm ball around the cheese. You should get about twenty-four arancini.
3. Spread the flour and bread crumbs on two rimmed plates. Beat the eggs in a shallow container. Dredge the arancini in the flour, tapping off the surplus. Immerse them in the beaten egg, allowing the surplus drip back into the container. Roll in bread crumbs to coat completely.
4. In a big straight-sided frying pan, heat 1 inch vegetable oil on moderate heat until the tip of an arancino sizzles on contact. Fry arancini in batches, taking care not to crowd the frying pan, turning on all sides, until golden, approximately 3 minutes per batch. Drain over paper towels, and sprinkle with salt while still warm.

Lemon-Rice Soup

Prep Time — 10 min

Cook Time — 16 min

Servings — 4

INGREDIENTS

- 5 cups Meat, Chicken, or Vegetable Broth, or 5 cups water plus 2 bouillon cubes and 1 tablespoon unsalted butter
- 1/2 cup Arborio rice
- 3 large eggs
- Juice of 1 lemon
- Salt to taste

DIRECTIONS

1. Place the broth (or water, bouillon cubes, and butter) in a large stockpot and bring to a boil over high heat. Add the rice, reduce the heat to medium, and simmer, checking the rice for doneness after 16 minutes. Rice should be al dente, or firm to the bite; do not overcook.
2. Beat the eggs with the lemon juice and season lightly with salt.
3. When the rice is just done, stir the eggs into the soup and serve immediately.

Rice

Rice with Olives

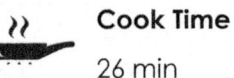

Prep Time 15 min **Cook Time** 26 min **Servings** 4

INGREDIENTS

- 2 large red bell peppers
- 1 cup dry white wine
- 1 large pinch saffron
- 1 tablespoon tomato paste
- 4 tablespoons olive oil
- 1 tablespoon unsalted butter
- 1 medium onion, minced
- 1 small whole fresh chili pepper
- 2 cups Arborio rice
- 2 hot Italian sausages (about 9 ounces)
- 20 pitted black olives, quartered
- Freshly ground black pepper to taste
- 2 quarts hot Meat Broth
- Preheat the oven to 350°F.

DIRECTIONS

1. Wash the bell peppers, then halve them and remove the seeds and any white pith. Cut the peppers into julienne and arrange them in a single layer on a large baking sheet. Place the peppers in the oven and roast 10 minutes, or until the peppers are wilted.
2. Remove the peppers from the oven and set aside. Place the wine in a small non-metallic bowl, add the saffron and tomato paste, and set aside.
3. Place the olive oil and the butter in a large Dutch oven over medium-low heat. When the butter is foamy, add the onion and the chili pepper and sauté gently until the onion is wilted but not browned, about 2 minutes.
4. Add the rice and stir to coat with the oil. Let stand 2 to 3 minutes, then add the sausage, olives, and wine mixture. Increase the heat to medium and simmer approximately 2 minutes, or until the wine has evaporated. Season to taste with black pepper and add the broth. Cover the Dutch oven, reduce the heat to low, and let cook 12 minutes, or until the rice is done—al dente, or firm to the bite.
5. When the rice is done, remove from the heat and spoon onto a large platter. Scatter the roasted red peppers over the top and serve immediately.

Basil Rice

Prep Time 15 min **Cook Time** 18 min **Servings** 4

INGREDIENTS

- 12 oz. (350 g) spaghetti.
- 2 1/4 lbs. (1 kg) clams, rubbed.
- 6 3/4 tbsp. (100 ml) extra-virgin olive oil.
- 1 tbsp. sliced fresh parsley.
- 1 clove garlic, cut.
- Salt and pepper.

DIRECTIONS

1. Bring a pot of well-salted water to a boil.
2. Warmth 1 tablespoon. Of oil in a huge frying pan. Include clams, cover, and chef up until they open up, 2-3 minutes get rid of frying pan from warm. Get rid of a few of clams from their coverings, pressure cooking liquid, and afterwards pour it back into skillet with clams. Allotted.
3. In another skillet, warmth continuing to be oil until hot. Include garlic and also chef till browned. Add clams and also their liquid as well as give a boil.
4. Meanwhile, prepare spaghetti in boiling water up until al dente. Drainpipe, scheduling some of pasta water. Include pasta to calm combination, adding a little pasta water if you want a wetter dish. Transfer to pasta bowls as well as serve, sprayed generously with pepper and also parsley.

Italian Cookbook 2022

Rice Cake

Prep Time: 20 min
Cook Time: 45 min
Servings: 8

INGREDIENTS

- 2 cups milk
- Salt to taste
- 1 1/2 cups Arborio rice
- 2 tablespoons unsalted butter
- 5 tablespoons freshly grated Parmesan cheese
- 4 large eggs, separated
- Freshly ground black pepper to taste

DIRECTIONS

1. Place the milk and salt in a large lidded saucepan and bring to a boil over high heat. Add the rice, cover, and reduce the heat to low. Let cook 15 minutes, stirring occasionally, until the liquid has been absorbed and the rice is al dente, or firm to the bite.
2. Remove the rice from the heat and stir in 1 tablespoon of the butter, the Parmesan cheese, and the egg yolks. Stir to combine thoroughly and season to taste with pepper. Set aside.
3. Preheat the oven to 350°F. Coat the inside of a 1 1/2-quart baking dish with the remaining 1 tablespoon butter.
4. Beat the egg whites thoroughly with a whisk or electric mixer until stiff but not dry. Fold the beaten whites into the rice and spoon the mixture into the prepared dish.
5. Place the dish in the oven and bake 30 minutes, or until the top of the rice cake is golden. Remove from the oven and loosen the edges of the cake with a knife. Invert the rice cake onto a platter and serve immediately.

NUTRITION: Calories: 369 | Fat: 16 g | Carbs: 44 g | Protein: 21.1 g | Cholesterol: 42 g

Cold Rice in Aspic

Prep Time: 25 min
Cook Time: 40 min
Servings: 4

INGREDIENTS

- 1 medium yellow bell pepper
- 1 medium red bell pepper
- 1 envelope unflavored gelatin
- 2 cups water
- 1 1/2 cups Marsala wine
- 2 cups Arborio rice
- 5 small fresh shrimp
- 1 hard-boiled egg, thinly sliced
- 15 pitted green olives, halved
- 1 6 1/2-ounce can tuna in olive oil, drained and flaked
- Juice of 1 lemon
- Salt to taste
- Freshly ground black pepper to taste
- 3 tablespoons olive oil

DIRECTIONS

1. Preheat the oven to 300°F. Cover a large baking sheet with aluminum foil.
2. Wash the peppers, then halve them and remove the seeds. Cut each half into julienne. Spread the pepper strips over the baking sheet and roast in the oven until wilted, about 10 minutes. Remove from the oven and allow to cool.
3. Dissolve the gelatin in the water and set aside to soften, about 10 minutes. Stir in the Marsala, then pour the mixture into a 2-quart mold. Place in the refrigerator to allow the aspic to harden a little bit.
4. Bring 4 quarts lightly salted water to a boil in a large saucepan. Add the rice and cook, checking for doneness after approximately 16 minutes. Rice should be al dente, or firm to the bite; do not overcook. When the rice is done, remove from the heat, pour into a colander, and rinse with cool water. Set the rice aside to drain and cool completely.
5. Meanwhile, bring 1 quart water to a boil in a medium saucepan. Add the shrimp and cook until pink and just done, about 4 minutes. Drain the shrimp, then peel them when cool enough to handle.
6. Remove the aspic from the refrigerator. Place the egg slices on top of the aspic, along with the shrimp and olives, in an attractive pattern.
7. Place the rice in a large mixing bowl and add the peppers, tuna, lemon juice, salt, pepper, and olive oil. Toss gently to combine. Spoon the rice on top of the aspic and press very gently into the mold. Refrigerate for at least 1 hour.
8. To serve, submerge the mold up to the rim in hot water for 1 or 2 minutes, then remove from the water and invert onto a serving platter.

Hot Rice Salad

Prep Time: 15 min
Cook Time: 20 min
Servings: 4

INGREDIENTS
- 2 cups Arborio rice
- 2 to 3 tablespoons olive oil
- Juice of 2 lemons
- 1/2 cup minced fresh parsley

DIRECTIONS
1. Bring 4 quarts lightly salted water to a boil in a large saucepan. Add the rice and cook, checking for doneness after approximately 16 minutes. Rice should be al dente, or firm to the bite; do not overcook. When the rice is done, remove from the heat and pour into a colander. Toss and press down gently to remove excess water, then transfer the rice immediately to a large serving platter.
2. Drizzle the olive oil and lemon juice over the hot rice and top with the parsley. Serve at once.

Italian Rice Pie

Prep Time: 20 min
Cook Time: 1 hour
Servings: 8

INGREDIENTS
- 9 large eggs eggs
- 1 ½ cups white sugar
- 2 pounds ricotta cheese
- 1 teaspoon vanilla extract
- 2 cups heavy whipping cream
- 1 cup cooked white rice
- 1 (15 ounce) can crushed pineapple, drained

DIRECTIONS
1. Whisk together the eggs in a large mixing bowl. Mix in the sugar thoroughly. Stir in the cheese and vanilla extract until the mixture is smooth and creamy. Stir in the heavy cream. Combine cooked rice and crushed pineapple in a mixing bowl.
2. Pour into a buttered 9 x 13-inch baking pan.
3. Preheat oven to 327.5°F (165°C) and bake for one hour.
4. Insert a clean knife into the center to check. The knife will be almost perfectly clean when the pie is done. The cake's top should be golden brown. Refrigerate until the mixture has completely chilled.

Nutrition:Calories 646.2 Cal | Protein 22g | Carbohydrates 59.3g | Fat 36.7g | Cholesterol 326mg | Sodium 244mg

Italian Rice with Porcini mushrooms

Prep Time: 20 min
Cook Time: 1 hour
Servings: 6

INGREDIENTS
- 2 cups beef broth, diluted with 2 cups water
- 2 tbsp. butter
- 2 tbsp. olive oil
- 2 tbsp. shallot, finely diced
- 1 clove garlic, finely diced
- 2 cups Arborio rice
- 1 package dry porcini mushrooms, about 1 oz
- Freshly ground black pepper
- 1/3 cup parmesan, freshly grated

DIRECTIONS
1. Soak the mushrooms in 2 cups of warm water, about 30 minutes to reconstitute. Squeeze mushrooms into the soaking juice once or twice while soaking. Remove from liquid. To eliminate any dirt, strain the liquid using a paper towel. Reserve. Chop mushrooms.
2. In a large pot, bring the broth to a simmer. Meanwhile, sauté shallot and garlic in half the butter and olive oil, about 5 minutes. Add the rice, and stir to coat. Next, add the first half cup of beef broth, stirring often. Add the mushrooms and 1 cup of the soaking water after 10 minutes. Cook until liquid has evaporated. Next, add the second half of the soaking liquid. Repeat the process until all water and broth have been incorporated, and rice is tender.
3. Remove from heat and season with pepper. Add 1 tablespoon butter and parmesan cheese. Adjust salt to taste and serve.

Milanese-Style Risotto

Prep Time 10 min   **Cook Time** 23 min   **Servings** 6

INGREDIENTS

- 5 cups Chicken Broth
- 2 tablespoons olive oil
- 1 small onion, minced
- 2 cups Arborio rice
- 1 large pinch of saffron
- Salt to taste
- Freshly ground black pepper to taste
- 1 1/2 tablespoons unsalted butter or margarine
- 4 tablespoons freshly grated Parmesan cheese

DIRECTIONS

1. Place the broth in a covered saucepan over high heat. When the broth is hot but not yet simmering, reduce the heat to low.
2. Place the olive oil in a large Dutch oven over medium heat. Add the onion and sauté gently until golden, about 3 minutes.
3. Add the rice and stir 1 to 2 minutes, or until the rice is well coated with oil.
4. Increase the heat to medium-high and add 1 cup of the hot broth, stirring constantly. When all of the broth has been absorbed by the rice, add another 1 cup broth and continue stirring.
5. Sprinkle in the saffron. Repeat the process as necessary for 16 minutes, or until the rice is al dente, or firm to the bite. Taste, and season with salt and pepper if needed.
6. Remove the risotto from the heat and stir in the butter and Parmesan cheese. Serve immediately.

Italian Rice with Saffron & Parmesan

Prep Time 20 min   **Cook Time** 35 min   **Servings** 6

INGREDIENTS

- 2 shallots, minced
- 1 clove garlic, minced
- 3 tbsp. olive oil
- 2 cups Arborio rice
- ½ tsp. saffron threads
- 6 cups chicken stock
- ½ cup dry white wine
- 1 cup fresh parmesan, grated finely, room temperature
- 4 tbsp. butter
- Freshly ground black pepper

DIRECTIONS

1. In a large saucepan, cook the shallots and garlic in olive oil until translucent, about 4–5 minutes. Stir in the rice, and cook an additional 3 minutes. Add the saffron threads, wine, and 2 cups of the stock. Bring to a simmer over medium heat. Cook, often stirring, until the majority of the liquid has been absorbed.
2. Remove the pan from the heat and stir in the parmesan cheese and 4 tablespoons butter. When each cup is incorporated chiefly, add a cup. Repeat until rice is thoroughly cooked.
3. Take the pan off the heat and add the parmesan and 4 tablespoons of butter. Add freshly ground black pepper to taste.

Rice with Potatoes and Leeks

Prep Time: 10 min | **Cook Time:** 20 min | **Servings:** 4

INGREDIENTS

- 13 1/3 oz. (350 g).Carnaroli rice.
- 3 1/2 oz. (100 g) unsalted butter.
- 3 oz. (80 g) mushrooms, thinly cut.
- 3 oz. (80 g) asparagus pointers.
- 3 oz. (80 g) Parma pork, cut into julienne.
- 3 oz. (80 g) peeled tomatoes, diced.
- 1/4 cup (5 cl) cream.
- 1/4 mugs (1 l) hot veal or beef stock.
- 3 oz. (80 g) grated Parmigiano-Reggiano cheese.
- 1/2 yellow onion, chopped.

1. Peel and dice potatoes.
2. Thaw butter in a Saucepan, and gently cook leeks. Include potatoes and also rice, and after that pour in broth a little each time. cook, mixing regularly and also adding more brew as it gradually comes to be absorbed. season to taste with Salt and pepper as well as offer.

Creamy Rice with Porcini

Prep Time: 12 min | **Cook Time:** 15 min | **Servings:** 4

INGREDIENTS

- ½ cup dry white wine
- ½ cup freshly grated Grana Padano
- ½ teaspoon kosher salt
- 1 cup minced onion
- 12 ounces fresh porcini mushrooms, thickly cut
- 2 cups Arborio or Carnaroli rice
- 2 tablespoons minced shallots
- 2 tablespoons unsalted butter, cut into bits
- 5 tablespoons extra-virgin olive oil
- 6½ cups hot Chicken Stock or Vegetable Stock
- Freshly ground black pepper to taste

DIRECTIONS

1. Bring the stock to a bare simmer in a moderate-sized deep cooking pan. Heat 3 tablespoons of the olive oil in a moderate-sized Dutch oven or big straight-sided frying pan, and sauté the onion and shallots until golden. Put in the mushrooms, and sauté until soft, approximately five minutes. Remove mushrooms, and save for later.
2. To the same pan put in the rest of the olive oil and the rice. Cook and stir to coat the rice with oil, until toasted but not colored, approximately three minutes. Pour in the wine, and cook until vaporized, approximately two minutes.
3. Put in ½ cup of the hot stock and the salt. Cook while stirring continuously, until all the liquid has been absorbed. Carry on to put in hot stock in small batches (barely sufficient to moisten the rice completely), stirring continuously to help the liquid absorb, until the rice mixture is creamy and firm to the bite. With the final addition of the stock, return the mushrooms to the pot, and stir and cook for another three to four minutes. Take the risotto from the heat, beat in the butter and then the cheese, flavor with pepper to taste, and serve instantly

---

Italian Jasmine Rice

Prep Time: 10 min | **Cook Time:** 5 min | **Servings:** 4

INGREDIENTS

- Salt and black pepper to the taste
- ¼ cup pine nuts
- 3 tablespoons butter
- 1 cup jasmine rice
- 2 tablespoons chives, chopped
- 2 teaspoons lemon juice

DIRECTIONS

1. Cook rice according to package instructions, fluff with a fork and leave aside for now.
2. Heat up a pan with the butter over medium high heat, add pine nuts, stir and brown for 3 minutes.
3. Add chives, lemon juice, rice, salt and pepper, stir, cook for 2 minutes more, divide between plates and serve.

NUTRITION: Calories: 280 Calories | Fiber: 1 g | Carbs: 34 g | Protein: 5g | Fat: 14 g

Soups

Lentil Soup

Prep Time 10 min **Cook Time** 30 min **Servings** 4

INGREDIENTS

- 1 cup dried lentils
- 1 small onion, finely diced
- 2 tablespoons chopped fresh parsley
- 2 or 3 carrots, peeled and thinly sliced
- 1 celery stalk, thinly sliced
- 3 tablespoons olive oil
- 1 teaspoon salt
- 1 (8-ounce) can tomatoes
- 3 cups Quick Vegetable Broth, or ½ large bouillon cube dissolved in 3 cups boiling water
- Water

DIRECTIONS

1. In a large bowl filled with cold water, soak the lentils for 1 hour.
2. In a large soup pot over medium-low heat, combine the onion, parsley, carrots, celery, oil, and salt, and sauté for several minutes until they become golden and fragrant.
3. Add the tomatoes and simmer for an additional minute.
4. Add the lentils, broth, and enough water to fully cover all the ingredients.
5. Simmer the soup over medium heat for 20 to 25 minutes until the lentils are fully cooked.

Garden Minestrone Soup

Prep Time 10 min **Cook Time** 35 min **Servings** 8

INGREDIENTS

- 4 medium carrots, chopped
- 1 medium zucchini, sliced
- 1/4 cup chopped onion
- 1 garlic clove, minced
- 1 tablespoon olive oil
- 2 cans (14-1/2 ounces each) vegetable broth
- 3 cups V8 juice
- 1 can (15 ounces) garbanzo beans or chickpeas, drained
- 1 can (14-1/2 ounces) diced tomatoes, undrained
- 1 cup frozen cut green beans
- 1/2 cup uncooked elbow macaroni
- 1 teaspoon dried basil
- 1 tablespoon minced fresh parsley

DIRECTIONS

1. Add the garlic, onion, zucchini and carrots into a Dutch oven, cook in oil until onion gets tender, or for 7 minutes. Add the basil, macaroni, green beans, tomatoes, garbanzo beans, V8 juice and broth. Boil them up.
2. Lower the heat, let it simmer while uncovering for 15 minutes. Mix in parsley. Cook for 5 more minutes or until macaroni gets tender.

NUTRITION: Calories: 166 Calories | Protein: 6g protein | Diabetic Exchanges: 3 vegetable | Total Fat: 3g fat (0 saturated fat) | Sodium: 900mg sodium | Fiber: 5g fiber) | Total Carbohydrate: 30g carbohydrate (0 sugars) | Cholesterol: 0 cholesterol

Italian Beef Stew

Prep Time 25 min **Cook Time** 90 min **Servings**

INGREDIENTS

- 4 pound Beef Chuck, cut into 2 1/2 " cubes
- 1 cup Flour
- ¼ teaspoon each Salt & Black Pepper
- 7 tablespoons Olive Oil
- 2 medium Onions, peeled and diced
- 2 tablespoons Butter
- 5 Carrots, peeled and cut into large dice
- 4 Idaho Potatoes, peeled and cut into large dice
- 2 ounce Dry Porcini Mushrooms, washed
- 2 cups dry Red Wine
- ½ can Tomato Paste
- Water
- 4 Garlic Cloves, peeled and sliced thin

DIRECTIONS

1. Place a few tablespoons of Olive Oil in a large pot that you will make the stew in. Turn heat on to high. Place the half of the beef in pot and brown over medium to high heat until all the beef is nicely browned, about 12 minutes. When browning the beef to not crowd, this is why you will brown the meat in 2 or 3 batches. When you brown the first batch of beef, set aside on a platter and finish browning all the beef.
2. Add the onions to pot with butter and cook over low heat for 5 minutes while stirring with a wooden spoon.
3. Add half the wine to pot and turn heat to high. You should have little brown bits sticking to the bottom of the pot from the browning of the beef which is what will give the stew a lot of its flavor. Stir the wine and onions and scrape the bottom of the pot so the brown bits incorporate into the wine. This is called deglazing. Cook until the wine has reduce by half its volume.
4. Add all the browned beef into the large pot with the onions and wine. Add remaining wine and cook over high heat until the liquid is reduce by half.
5. Add the tomato paste and water to cover the beef slightly.
6. Cook over high heat until the liquid comes to the boil. Once it comes to the boil, lower heat so the liquid is at a light simmer.
7. As the stew is simmering, put the Dry Porcini Mushrooms in warm water to cover and let soak for 15 minutes. Add to pot after the stew has been simmering for 1 hour. Make sure to stir from time to time with a wooden spoon, scraping the bottom of the pot so the stew doesn't burn.
8. After the stew has been simmering for 1 hour and a half, add carrots to pot and continue cooking at a low simmer.
9. After stew has been simmering for 2 hours add the potatoes and continue cooking until the potatoes are cooked and the beef is tend, about 35 minutes. The stew is now finished.
10. Taste a bit of the liquid to see if you have to adjust the seasoning by adding a bit more Salt and or Pepper or not.
11. Serve in shallow soup bowls and save leftover stew in air-tight containers to enjoy at another meal.

Basil Spaghetti Soup

Prep Time 15 min **Cook Time** 12 min **Servings** 4

- 1 cup spaghetti, cooked
- 1 tsp. garlic, chopped
- 1 cup carrots & French beans, chopped
- 1/2 cup onions, chopped
- 2 tsp. olive oil
- 6 cups vegetable stock
- A few drops of tabasco sauce
- 8 basil leaves, chopped
- Salt and ground black pepper, to taste

1. Oil the pan and add garlic and onions for 5 minutes.
2. Then, add salt, Tabasco sauce, pepper, and pasta. Bring to boil for 5 minutes.
3. Garnish with basil leaves. Serve hot.
4. Basil spaghetti soup is ready.

Chickpea Soup

Prep Time: 10 min   **Cook Time:** 20 min   **Servings:** 4

INGREDIENTS

- 3 tablespoons olive oil, plus more for drizzling
- ½ small onion, chopped
- 2 carrots, peeled and finely diced
- 1 (14-ounce) can diced tomatoes
- 4 cups Quick Vegetable Broth, or ½ large bouillon cube dissolved in 4 cups boiling water
- 2 cans chickpeas, drained and rinsed
- 12 ounces fresh spinach
- Salt
- Freshly ground black pepper

DIRECTIONS

1. In a large stockpot, heat the oil over medium heat.
2. Add the onion and carrots, and sauté for several minutes until the vegetables soften slightly. Add the tomatoes.
3. Add the broth and enough water to fill the pan a bit past the halfway mark. Bring the soup to a full boil.
4. Once the broth is boiling, add the chickpeas and spinach, and simmer for 15 minutes.
5. Add salt and pepper to taste and drizzle with additional oil, if desired.

Nutrition: Calories 356 Cal | Fats 12.2 g | Sodium: 585 mg | Carbohydrates 46.8 g | Protein 18.2 g

Recipe Italian Wedding Soup

Prep Time: 20 min   **Cook Time:** 2 hours   **Servings:** 4

INGREDIENTS

- 8 cups water, 4 cups chicken broth
- 1 large onion, chopped. 2 carrots diced
- 1 head escarole, finely chopped
- ¾ lb. ground beef
- 3/4 lb. ground pork
- 1 cup grated Parmigiano,
- ¼ fresh parsley, finely chopped.
- 1 clove garlic, finely chopped
- 1 medium bay leaf
- 1-3 lb. broiler chicken,
- 6 cloves garlic, peeled

DIRECTIONS

1. Season with salt and pepper and combine ground meat, eggs, parsley, minced garlic, and Parmigiano-Reggiano. Form into marble-sized meatballs. Then set aside.
2. In a large pot, bring the whole chicken, whole garlic, bay leaf, and water to a boil. Reduce flame to a lower heat and cook for 1 hour and 15 minutes.
3. Place meatballs in a lightly oiled baking tray and bake for 8 minutes at 350 degrees.
4. Remove the chicken from the pot and leave it aside to cool. Simmer for another 12 minutes with the carrots and onions in the broth. Add the escarole and cook for 12 minutes at medium heat. Chicken meat should be removed from the bones and diced. Add the meatballs and diced chicken flesh to the stock and cook for 12 minutes on the lowest setting.

Serve the soup in dishes, with at least 5 small meatballs for each person. Pass the Mangia Bene and Parmigiano.

Note: You can substitute Sausage for the Meatballs, which is how some people make this soup. It's just as tasty and cuts down on some of the work. If doing so, substitute 1 /2 pounds of Italian Sweet Sausages for the meatballs. Lightly brown the links of sausage over low heat for 6 minutes. Remove from pan and cut each link into 6 equal size pieces, then add to soup in the same point (step 6) and cook over low heat in soup for 12 minutes.

Soups

Escarole and Bean Soup

Prep Time 20 min **Cook Time** 18 min **Servings**

- 4 tablespoons Olive Oil
- 1 medium Onion, peeled and minced
- 2 Carrots, peeled and minced fine
- 4 cloves Garlic, peeled and minced fine
- 2 cans Lite Chicken Broth
- 1 quart water, 1 Bay Leaf
- ½ teaspoon Sea Salt, ½ teaspoon Black Pepper
- 1 large head Escarole
- 2 cans Cannellini Beans, drain and wash the beans
- ¼ cup grated Parmigiano

1. Place olive oil, onions, and garlic in a 6-quart non-corrosive pot. Turn flame on low and cook for 5 minutes. Add carrots and continue cooking on low heat for 2 minutes.
2. Add Chicken Broth, water, Bay Leaf, Salt & Black Pepper and turn heat to high. Let boil for 6 minutes.
3. Cut bottom end off Escarole and discard. Cut the escarole into 1/12" strips. Wash escarole thoroughly.
4. Add escarole to pot and cook at a hard boil for 4 minutes.
5. Add cannellini beans to pot and cook on medium low heat for 8 minutes.
6. To serve, fill soup bowls with soup. Drizzle a little olive oil over top of soup, and pass around grated Parmigiano Reggiano or Pecorino Romano Cheese.

Sausage, Potato and Kale Soup

Prep Time 10 min **Cook Time** 25 min **Servings** 6

- 5 teaspoons olive oil
- 1 (16 ounce) package fettuccini pasta
- 4 shallots, diced
- 3 egg yolks
- 1 large onion, cut into thin strips
- 1/2 cup heavy cream
- 1 pound bacon, cut into strips
- 3/4 cup shredded Parmesan cheese
- 1 clove garlic, chopped
- salt and pepper to taste

1. In a big heavy saucepan, heat the olive oil over medium heat. Soften shallots in a skillet. Cook, stirring frequently, until the bacon is evenly browned. When the bacon is approximately halfway done, add the garlic. Remove the pan from the heat.
2. Boil a large saucepan of lightly salted water. Cook for 8 to 10 minutes, or until pasta is al dente. Return the spaghetti to the saucepan after draining it.
3. Whisk together egg yolks, cream, and shredded Parmesan in a medium mixing basin. Stir in the cream mixture after pouring the bacon mixture over the spaghetti. Salt & pepper to taste.

NUTRITION: Calories 614 | Protein 26 | Fat 28.6g | Cholesterol 166 mg | Sodium 498.1mg | Carbs: 64.8 g

Cream Of Tomato Soup

Prep Time 5 min **Cook Time** 20 min **Servings** 6

INGREDIENTS

- 2 tablespoons butter
- 1 onion, chopped
- 2 tablespoons all-purpose flour
- 1 quart tomato juice
- salt to taste
- 2 cups milk

DIRECTIONS

1. In a Dutch oven, sauté onions in melted butter over medium heat until translucent. Take away from the heat. Mix in the flour to get no lumps remained, and then slowly stir in the tomato juice. Take back to the heat and put in salt to taste. Cook until starting boiling, but turn off the heat before it boils. Allow to cool in 10 minutes, and then slowly mix in milk. Enjoy immediately.

NUTRITION: Calories: 119 Calories | Total Fat: 5.6 | Sodium: 494 | Total Carbohydrate: 14.3 | Cholesterol: 17 | Protein: 4.4

Italian Cookbook 2022

Garlic Tomato Soup

Prep Time 30 min **Cook Time** 30 min **Servings** 4

INGREDIENTS

- 12 garlic cloves, peeled and sliced
- 1-1/2 teaspoons olive oil
- 1 can (14-1/2 ounces) diced tomatoes, undrained
- 1 cup tomato puree
- 1 pint heavy whipping cream
- 1/4 teaspoon dried oregano
- 1/4 teaspoon minced fresh basil
- 1/4 teaspoon salt
- 1/8 teaspoon pepper

DIRECTIONS

1. Combine garlic and oil in a 3 cup baking dish. Cover then bake in the oven at 300 degrees until browned lightly, or for about 25 - 30 minutes.
2. Boil tomato puree, tomatoes, and garlic in a large saucepan. Lower the heat and simmer while covered for 30 minutes.
3. Add pepper, salt, basil, oregano, and cream, then slightly cool. In a blender, place 1/2 of the soup at a time, then cover and process until pureed. Return the soup onto the pan and heat through.

Nutrition: Calories 130 Cal | Fats 4 g | Sodium: 355 mg | Protein 6 g | Cholesterol: 9 mg | Fiber: 2 g | Carbs: 18 g

---

Slow Cooked Vegetable Soup

Prep Time 20 min **Cook Time** 9 hours **Servings** 12

INGREDIENTS

- 3/4 cup chopped onion
- 1/2 cup chopped celery
- 1/2 cup chopped green pepper
- 2 tablespoons olive oil
- 1 large potato, peeled and diced
- 1 medium sweet potato, peeled and diced
- 1 to 2 garlic cloves, minced
- 3 cups vegetable broth
- 2 medium fresh tomatoes, chopped
- 1 can (16 ounces) kidney beans, rinsed and drained
- 1 can (15 ounces) garbanzo beans or chickpeas, rinsed and drained
- 2 teaspoons soy sauce
- 1 teaspoon paprika
- 1/2 teaspoon dried basil
- 1/4 teaspoon salt
- 1/4 teaspoon ground turmeric
- 1 bay leaf
- Dash cayenne pepper

DIRECTIONS

In the big skillet, sauté green pepper, celery and onion in oil till crisp-tender. Put in the garlic, sweet potato and potato; sauté 3 to 5 more minutes. Place in the 5-quart slow cooker. Mix in rest ingredients. Keep it covered and cook over low heat till the veggies are softened or for 9 to 10 hours. Get rid of the bay leaf.

Nutrition: Calories: 136 Cal | Sodium: 449mg | Fiber: 5g | Total Carbohydrate: 22g | Protein: 6g | Total Fat: 3g

Soups

Braised Oxtail Stew

Prep Time: 20 min
Cook Time: 4 hours and 15 min
Servings: 6

INGREDIENTS

- 5 lb. oxtails, cut into pieces
- 1 bottle of red wine
- 2 cups beef broth
- Salt and pepper to taste
- 1 tsp. garlic powder
- 4 tbsp. butter
- 1 diced onion
- 4 minced garlic cloves
- 1 tsp. onion powder
- 1 tsp. tarragon
- 1 bay leaf
- 5 cups beef broth
- 2 cups sliced mushrooms
- 2 sliced carrots
- 2 peeled and cubed potatoes
- 3 tbsp. butter

DIRECTIONS

1. Preheat the oven to 325.
2. Season the oxtails with garlic and onion powders, salt, and pepper.
3. Melt 1 tbsp. Butter in a large pan and brown the oxtails for 10 minutes.
4. Transfer the oxtails to a platter.
5. Add another tbsp. Butter and sauté the onion and garlic for 5 minutes.
6. Add the tarragon, bay leaf, beef broth, and wine.
7. Place the saucepan in the oven, covered.
8. Cook for 3 hours.
9. Remove the cover with care and add the carrots, potatoes, and mushrooms.
10. Cook for about 45 minutes more, or until the veggies are tender.
11. Place the meat and vegetables in a dish.
12. Strain the liquid into a pot and cook on low until you are left with 2 cups of broth, about 20 minutes.
13. Add the butter and stir until it melts before pouring it over the meat and veggies.

Quick Italian Vegetable Soup

Prep Time: 15 min
Cook Time: 30 min
Servings: 6

INGREDIENTS

- 1 tablespoon olive oil
- 1 medium onion, chopped
- 2 thin strips carrots, sliced
- 2 stalks celery, sliced
- 1 (16 ounce) can diced plum tomatoes
- 2 teaspoons Italian seasoning
- 2 cubes beef bouillon
- 6 cups water
- 2 medium (blank)s zucchinis, quartered and sliced
- 2 cups sliced cabbage
- 1 teaspoon garlic salt
- 1 teaspoon salt and ground black pepper to taste
- ½ cup freshly grated Parmesan cheese

DIRECTIONS

1. In a large stockpot, heat the oil over medium-high heat. For 5-7 minutes, sauté onion, carrot, and celery until onion is transparent and vegetables are soft. Cook for another 5 minutes, stirring often, after adding the tomatoes and Italian spice.
2. In a small bowl, dissolve the bouillon cubes in water and stir them into the vegetables. Reduce the heat and simmer for about 10 minutes. Add the zucchini and cabbage, season with garlic salt, and simmer for another 5 minutes, or until soft. Season with salt and pepper, then serve.

NUTRITION: Calories 93 Cal | Protein 4.9g | Carbohydrates 10g | Fat 4.5g | Cholesterol 5.9mg | Sodium 1210.2mg |

Zucchini Tomato Soup

Prep Time: 10 min
Cook Time: 10 min
Servings: 6

INGREDIENTS

- 2 medium zucchinis, chopped
- 1/4 cup red onion, chopped
- 1/2 tablespoons olive oil
- 1/8 teaspoon salt
- 1 cup spicy hot V8 juice
- 1 tomato, cut into wedges
- Dash each pepper and dry basil
- 2 tbsp. shredded cheddar cheese (optional)
- 2 tbsp. crumbled cooked bacon (optional)

DIRECTIONS

1. Add onion and zucchini into a big skillet, sauté in oil until crisp tender. Scatter salt over, Add the basil, pepper, tomato and V8 juice; cook until heated through. Scatter bacon and cheese if preferred

Nutrition: Calories 89 Cal | Fats 4 g | Sodium: 545 mg | Protein 3 g | Fiber: 3 g | Carbs: 12 g

---

Fish stock

Prep Time: 15 min
Cook Time: 30 min
Servings: 2 1/2 quarts

INGREDIENTS

- 1 tablespoon extra-virgin olive oil
- 1 teaspoon black peppercorns
- 2 celery stalks, cut into big chunks
- 2 pounds fish heads and trimmings from nonoily fish, such as red snapper and sea bass (freshness is paramount, but frozen when fresh is fine)
- 2 small onions, halved
- 4 garlic cloves
- 4 medium carrots, peeled and cut into big chunks
- 6 sprigs fresh Italian parsley
- Kosher salt to taste

DIRECTIONS

1. Wash the fish heads and trimmings well using cool running water. Mix all of the ingredients apart from the salt in a big pot. Put in 4 quarts cold water. Bring to its boiling point, then simmer gently for an hour, skimming off and discarding the foam that rises to the surface.
2. Strain the stock through a twofold thickness of moistened cheesecloth. Flavor mildly with salt. This stock can be used instantly or placed in the fridge for maximum 2 days or frozen for maximum a month.

Soups

Mixed Meat Stock

Prep Time 20 min

Cook Time 3 hours and 25 min

Servings 2 quarts

INGREDIENTS

- 1 bunch Italian parsley, washed
- 1 medium onion
- 1 pound beef short ribs
- 1 pound chicken backs and wings
- 1 pound veal bones
- 2 big carrots, peeled and halved
- 2 celery stalks
- 4 peppercorns
- 4 whole garlic cloves
- Extra-virgin olive oil
- Kosher salt

DIRECTIONS

1. Preheat your oven to 425 degrees. Trim the meats of surplus fat, and wash. In a big roasting pan toss the meat and bones with olive oil. Roast until mildly browned, approximately twenty-five minutes.
2. Put the meat and bones in a big stockpot. Cover liberally with cold water (about 5 quarts), salt very lightly, and slowly bring to its boiling point.
3. In the same roasting pan, toss the vegetables with olive oil and roast until mildly browned, approximately twenty minutes. Put them into the stockpot with the parsley and peppercorns.
4. Simmer until dark and flavorful, approximately three to four hours, skimming froth and fat as they accumulate on the surface. Take off the stove, put in salt if required, strain through a very fine sieve, and place in your fridge overnight. The next day, skim off the solid surface fat. The stock then can be placed safely in the refrigerator for maximum three days or frozen for quite a few months.

Broccoli Soup

Prep Time 20 min

Cook Time 1 hour approx

Servings 2 quarts

INGREDIENTS

- ¼ cup extra-virgin olive oil
- 1 big head broccoli, florets chopped, stems peeled and chopped
- 2 bunches scallions, trimmed and chopped (about 2 cups)
- 2 garlic cloves, chopped
- 2 medium potatoes, peeled and chopped into 1-inch pieces (approximately 1¼ pounds)
- 2 ounces pancetta, finely diced
- 2 tablespoons tomato paste
- 2 teaspoons kosher salt
- Grated Pecorino Romano, for serving

DIRECTIONS

1. In a moderate-sized Dutch oven, heat the olive oil on moderate heat. When the oil is hot, put in the pancetta, and cook until the fat is rendered, approximately three minutes. Put in the garlic and potatoes, and cook, stirring once in a while, until potatoes start to stick to the bottom of the pan, approximately five minutes.
2. Make a spot in the bottom of the pan, and put in the tomato paste. Cook and stir the tomato paste in that spot until it toasts and darkens a shade or two, approximately two minutes. Put in 3 quarts water, and bring to its boiling point. Simmer, covered, until potatoes are soft, approximately fifteen minutes.
3. Put in the broccoli florets and stems, scallions, and salt. Simmer, uncovered, until the broccoli is soft, the florets have broken down, and the soup is thick and flavorful, approximately 35 minutes. Serve the soup with a drizzle of Pecorino Romano

Cauliflower and Tomato Soup

Prep Time 10 min **Cook Time** 10 min **Servings** 2.5 quarts

INGREDIENTS
- ¼ cup extra-virgin olive oil, plus more for drizzling
- ¼ cup tomato paste
- ½ cup chopped fresh Italian parsley
- ½ teaspoon crushed red pepper flakes
- 1 big carrot, peeled and chopped
- 1 big head cauliflower, cut into 1-inch pieces, including the tender leaves
- 1 medium onion, chopped
- 1 tablespoon chopped fresh thyme
- 1½ cups long-grain rice
- 2 fresh bay leaves
- 4 celery stalks, chopped
- 4 teaspoons kosher salt
- Freshly grated Grana Padano, for serving

DIRECTIONS

1. To a big Dutch oven on moderate heat, put in the olive oil. When the oil is hot, put in the onion, carrot, and celery. Cook until the vegetables start to soften, approximately five minutes. Clear a space in the pan and put in the tomato paste. Cook and stir the tomato paste in that spot until it is toasted and darkens a shade or two, approximately two to three minutes. Put in 5 quarts cold water, the bay leaves, thyme, crushed red pepper, and salt. Bring to its boiling point, and simmer quickly, uncovered, until vegetables are soft, approximately half an hour.
2. Put in the cauliflower, cover, and cook until the cauliflower is super soft, approximately half an hour.
3. Put in the rice. Uncover and simmer quickly until the soup is thickened and the rice is just tender, approximately fifteen minutes. (If you are not going to serve all of the soup at once, just cook the rice in the amount of soup you want to serve, and chop the rice proportionally.)
4. Remove bay leaves. Put in the parsley, and serve soup with a sprinkle of olive oil and a drizzle of grated cheese.

Tuscan Bean Soup

Prep Time 10 min **Cook Time** 25 min **Servings** 4

INGREDIENTS
- 3 tablespoons olive oil
- 2 carrots, peeled and diced
- 1 small onion, diced
- 3 tablespoons chopped fresh parsley
- 3 hot Italian sausages, cut into 5 pieces
- 1 8oz-can diced tomatoes
- 2 15oz-can cannellini beans, rinsed and drained
- Salt to taste

DIRECTIONS

1. Combine the oil, carrots, onion, and parsley in a large soup pot. Sauté for 2 to 3 minutes, or until the color has developed, but they are still crisp. Add the sausage and brown it on all sides with a wooden spoon for 2 to 3 minutes.
2. Continue to sauté for another 2 to 3 minutes after adding the tomatoes. Add the beans and just enough water to cover everything—season with salt to taste.
3. Bring to a boil, then reduce to low heat and cook for another 20 minutes, or until the beans are thoroughly cooked.

Soups

Italian Potato Soup

Prep Time 10 min | **Cook Time** 25 min | **Servings** 4

INGREDIENTS

- 3 tablespoons olive oil
- 1 large onion, chopped
- 5 cups water
- 4 medium (2-1/4" to 3" dia, raw)s potatoes, peeled and quartered
- salt and pepper to taste
- 4 large eggs

DIRECTIONS

1. Heat the oil in a large pot over medium heat. Cook onions until they are translucent. Add water, potatoes, salt, and pepper to the onions. Bring to a boil, then reduce to a low heat and continue to cook for 20 minutes, or until potatoes are cooked but firm.
2. Remove the pan from the heat and carefully crack the eggs into the soup, being careful not to break them. Cook over low heat until the egg whites are done. Before serving, allow it cool somewhat

NUTRITION: Calories 342 Cal | Protein 10.3g | Carbohydrates 42.2g | Fat 15.3g | Cholesterol 186mg | Sodium 531.4mg

---

Rice and Potato Soup

Prep Time 20 min | **Cook Time** 1 hour | **Servings** 8

INGREDIENTS

- ¼ cup freshly grated Grana Padano
- ½ cup chopped fresh Italian parsley
- 1 cup long-grain rice
- 2 big russet potatoes, peeled and cut into 1-inch cubes
- 2 center celery stalks, trimmed and diced
- 2 fresh bay leaves
- 2 medium carrots, trimmed, peeled, and coarsely shredded
- 2 teaspoons tomato paste
- 3 tablespoons extra-virgin olive oil
- Freshly ground black pepper
- Kosher salt
- Leftover rind of Grana Padano cheese, washed

DIRECTIONS

1. In a big soup pot, heat the olive oil on moderate heat. Put in the potatoes, and cook, stirring once in a while, until mildly browned, approximately five minutes. (It's fine if the potatoes stick; just adjust the level of heat to prevent the bits of potato that stick from getting too dark.)
2. Mix in the carrots and celery, and cook, stirring using a wooden spoon, until the carrots become tender, approximately two to three minutes. Flavor mildly with salt, then mix in the tomato paste to coat the vegetables. Pour in 10 cups water and put in the bay leaves, then bring to its boiling point, scraping up the bits of stuck potato.
3. Put in the cheese rind, adjust the level of heat to keep soup at a simmer, and season the soup lightly with salt and pepper. Cover the pot, and simmer until the potatoes start to fall apart, approximately forty minutes.
4. Mix the rice into the hot soup and let simmer, stirring well, until the rice is soft but still firm, approximately twelve minutes.
5. Take the bay leaves and the cheese rind. Drizzle the parsley into the soup, and flavor with the grated cheese and salt and pepper to taste.

Roman "Egg Drop" Soup

Prep Time: 15 min | **Cook Time:** 20 min | **Servings:** 6

INGREDIENTS
- 1/3 cup freshly grated Grana Padano, plus more for serving
- 1¼ teaspoons kosher salt
- 4 big eggs
- 4 cups packed spinach leaves, shredded
- 8 cups defatted homemade Chicken Stock
- Freshly ground black pepper

DIRECTIONS
1. In a moderate-sized pot, bring the stock to a simmer. Once it is simmering, put in 1 teaspoon salt and the spinach and cook until soft, approximately three minutes.
2. In the meantime, in a moderate-sized bowl, whisk together eggs, grated cheese, rest of the ¼ teaspoon salt, and some freshly ground black pepper to taste.
3. Once the spinach is soft, put in about a third of the egg mixture to the soup, while constantly whisking the soup where the egg is falling, to make shreds of the eggs. Put in and whisk rest of the eggs in two more batches, allowing the soup to return to its boiling point between additions. Once all of the eggs have been added, bring soup to a final boil, and use the whisk to break up any big clusters of eggs. Serve soup with additional grated cheese.

Bell Pasta Soup

Prep Time: 10 min | **Cook Time:** 20 min | **Servings:** 8

- 1 tbsp olive oil
- 1 onion, chopped
- 2 cloves garlic, minced
- 1 red bell pepper, chopped
- 3 C. low fat, low chicken broth
- 1 C. canned whole tomatoes, chopped
- 1 1/2 C. kidney beans, cooked
- 2 tsps chopped fresh thyme
- 1/2 C. chopped spinach
- 1 C. seashell pasta
- ground black pepper to taste

1. Place a large pot on medium heat. Heat the oil in it. Add the onion and garlic then cook them for 5 min. Stir in the bell pepper and cook them for 3 min.
2. Stir in the broth, tomatoes and beans. Cook them until they start boiling. Lower the heat and simmer the soup for 20 min.
3. Add the thyme, spinach and pasta. Cook the soup for 5 min. Adjust the seasoning of the soup. Serve it warm. Enjoy.

NUTRITION: Calories 174 kcal | Fat:3.1 g | Carbohydrates:29g | Protein 8 g | Cholesterol: 0 mg | Sodium :409 mg

Beef Soup

Prep Time: 10 min | **Cook Time:** 40-60 min | **Servings:** 4

- 2 teaspoons salt, or more
- 3 carrots, peeled and diced into 2-inch pieces
- 2 celery stalks, cut into 5 to 7 pieces
- 1 large onion, quartered
- Small handful parsley sprigs, stemmed
- 1 cup diced fresh or canned tomatoes
- 2 pounds various cuts of beef

1. Put all the ingredients in a large soup pot. Add enough water to fill the pot to a few inches below the top.
2. Boil the soup for 40 minutes to 1 hour, depending on the cuts of beef used. Tender cuts will take closer to 40 minutes, while tougher cuts will take closer to 1 hour. Skim off any beef fat that rises to the top.
3. Serve this soup as a first course. You can also strain and discard all the non-meat ingredients, chop up the meat, and serve just the broth and the meat.

Nutrition: Calories 465 Cal | Fat 14.3g | Carbs 10 g | Protein 70.1 g | Sodium: 1354 mg

Soups

Smokey Mediter- Soup

Prep Time 10 min

Cook Time 40 min

Servings 4

INGREDIENTS

- 1 garlic clove, minced
- 2 garlic cloves, sliced
- 2 teaspoons thyme, chopped
- 1 egg, whisked
- 12 ounces pork meat, ground
- 12 ounces veal, ground
- Salt and black pepper to the taste
- 3 ounces manchego, grated
- A pinch of saffron
- 15 ounces canned tomatoes, crushed
- 2 tablespoons extra virgin olive oil
- 1/3 cup panko
- 4 cups chicken stock
- 1 tablespoons parsley, chopped
- 8 ounces pasta

DIRECTIONS

1. In a bowl, mix veal with pork, 1 garlic clove, 1 teaspoon thyme, ¼ teaspoon paprika, salt, pepper to the taste, egg, manchego a panko and stir very well.
2. Shape 20 meatballs from this mix using your wet hands and put them on a plate.
3. Heat up a pan with 1 and ½ tablespoons oil over medium high heat, add half of the meatballs, cook for 2 minutes on each side, transfer to paper towels, drain grease and put on a plate.
4. Repeat this with the rest of the meatballs.
5. Heat up the pot with the rest of the oil, add sliced garlic, stir and cook for 1 minute.
6. Add the rest of the thyme, the rest of the paprika, saffron, stock and tomatoes, stir and cook for 2 minutes.
7. Add meatballs, stir, reduce heat to medium low, cook for 25 minutes and season with salt and pepper.
8. Cook pasta is accruing to instructions, drain them, put into a bowl and mix with ½ cup soup.
9. Divide pasta into soup bowls, add soup and meatballs on top, sprinkle parsley all over and serve.

Nutrition: Calories 380 Cal | Fat 17g | Fiber 2g | Carbohydrates 28g | Protein 26g

Italian Halibut Chowder

Prep Time 20 min

Cook Time 1 hour and 10 min

Servings 8

INGREDIENTS

- 2 1/4 lb. cubed halibut steaks
- 1 red bell pepper, chopped
- 1 onion, chopped
- 3 stalks celery, chopped
- 3 cloves garlic, minced
- ¼ cup olive oil
- 1 cup tomato juice
- ½ cup apple juice
- 2 16oz. cans whole peeled tomatoes, mashed
- 2 tbsp. chopped fresh parsley
- ½ teaspoon salt
- ½ teaspoon dried basil
- ⅛ teaspoon dried thyme
- A pinch of freshly ground black pepper

DIRECTIONS

1. In a skillet, cook the peppers, celery, onion, and garlic until soft. Combine the tomato juice or water, apple juice, mashed tomatoes, and herbs in a large mixing bowl—Cook for 30 minutes on low heat.
2. Toss the halibut pieces into the soup. Cook for 30 minutes or until the halibut is done. Season with salt and pepper to taste.

NUTRITION: Calories: 263 | Calories | Total Fat: 10.3 g | Sodium: 399.7 g | Carbs: 10.7 g | Cholesterol: 17 | Protein: 31.2 g

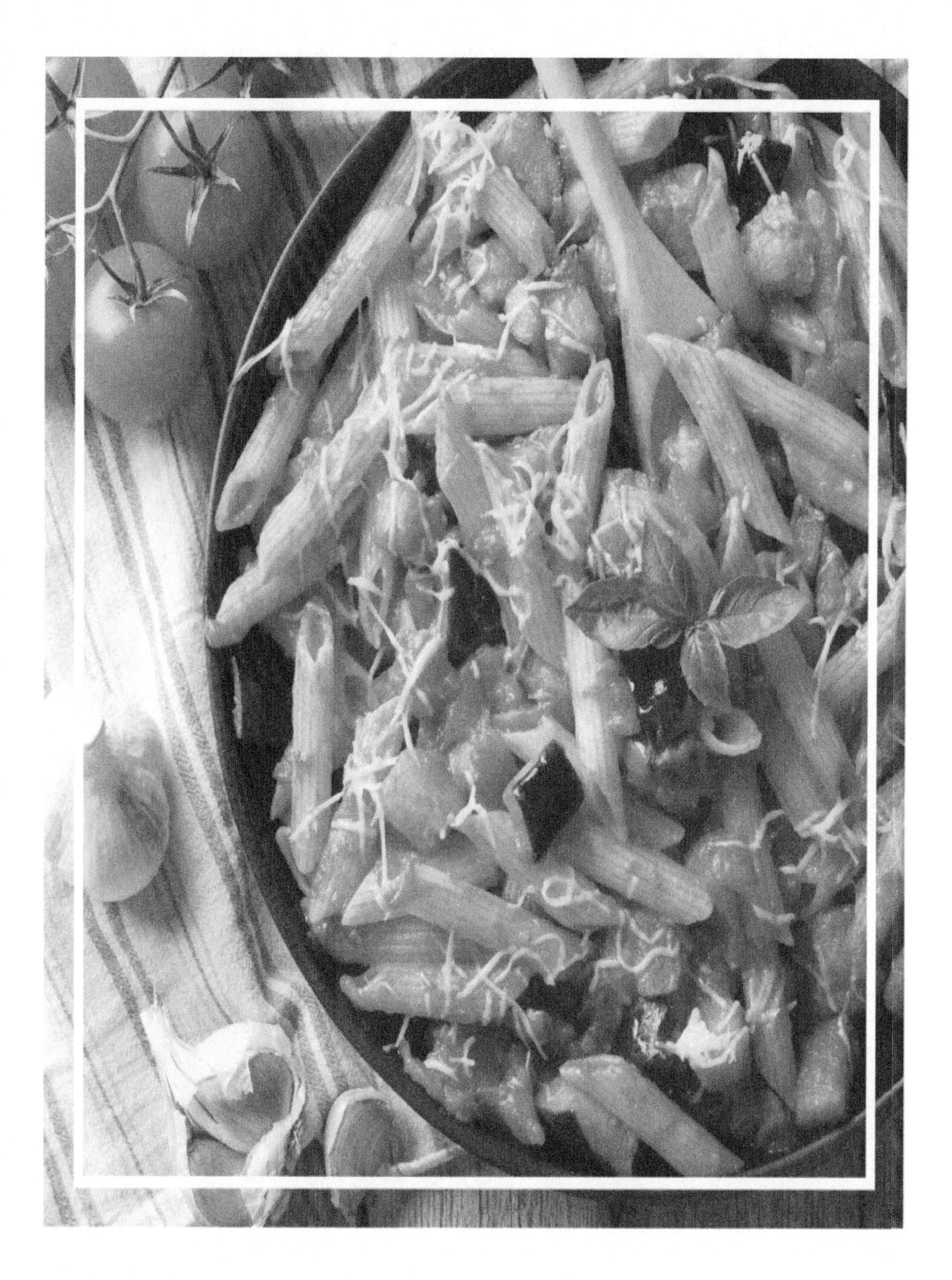

Bread and Pizza

Pizza Dough

Prep Time: 1 hour and 30 min
Cook Time: 0 min
Servings: 4

INGREDIENTS

- 100 g of Strong Flour
- 165 g of Whole meal Flour
- 135 ml of water
- 8 g of active yeast
- ½ teaspoon of malt (about 2 g)
- 1 teaspoon of EVO oil (about 5 g)
- 1 teaspoon of salt (about 5 g)

DIRECTIONS

1. Start dissolving 8 g of yeast in 135 ml of water together with 1/2 teaspoon of malt.
2. Add 100 g of strong flour, 165 g of whole meal flour and start kneading;
3. After a few minutes, add 1 teaspoon of salt, 1 teaspoon of oil and continue to knead until you reach the dough point;
4. Let the dough rest for 20 minutes;
5. Divide it into two equal parts and form two balls;
6. Let them rise for 5/6 hours in a sealed container at room temperature;
7. When the dough is doubled, you can proceed with the stretching, topping, and cooking.

Italian Herbed Pizza Dough

Prep Time: 20 min
Cook Time: 1 hour and 40 min
Servings: 4 pizza doughs

INGREDIENTS

- 1 package active dry yeast
- 1½ cups warm water (about 110°F)
- 2 tablespoons extra-virgin olive oil
- 3 garlic cloves, minced
- 1 teaspoon dried oregano
- ½ teaspoon dried basil
- ½ teaspoon onion powder
- 4 cups all-purpose flour, plus more for dusting
- 1½ teaspoons salt

DIRECTIONS

1. In a medium bowl, add the yeast to the warm water and let bloom for about 10 minutes. Add the olive oil, garlic, oregano, basil, and onion powder.
2. In a food processor, pulse to blend the flour and salt. With the machine running, add the yeast mixture in a slow, steady stream. Turn the machine off as soon as the dough comes together. Turn the dough out onto a well-floured board and, with lightly floured hands, knead the dough using the heels of your hands, pushing the dough and then folding it over. Shape into a ball and cut into 2 or 4 pieces.
3. Place the balls on a lightly floured pan and cover with a kitchen towel. Let the dough rise until it doubles in volume, about 1½ hours.

Shaved Asparagus, Ricotta, and Oven-roasted Tomato Pizza

Prep Time: 20 min **Cook Time:** 50 min **Servings:** 4

INGREDIENTS

- 4 tomatoes, cut into ¼-inch-thick slices
- ½ teaspoon salt
- 1 tablespoon extra-virgin olive oil
- 3 tablespoons balsamic vinegar, divided

For the pizza:
- Cornmeal or flour, for dusting
- 1 tablespoon extra-virgin olive oil, plus more for brushing
- 1 pound asparagus, shaved into long ribbons with a vegetable peeler
- 1 lemon wedge, for squeezing
- ¼ cup grated Parmesan cheese
- ¼ teaspoon fine sea salt
- ⅛ teaspoon freshly ground black pepper
- Italian-Herbed Pizza Dough
- ½ cup ricotta cheese

DIRECTIONS

To make the oven-roasted tomatoes:
1. Preheat the oven and pizza stone (if using) to 275°F. Line a baking sheet with foil.
2. Spread the tomatoes on the prepared baking sheet. Season with the salt, and drizzle with the olive oil and 1½ tablespoons of balsamic vinegar. Transfer to the oven and roast for 20 minutes, or until the tomatoes have collapsed.
3. Drizzle the remaining 1½ tablespoons of balsamic vinegar over the tomatoes, and continue cooking for 20 minutes more, or until they are caramelized. Remove the baking sheet from the oven and transfer the tomatoes to a medium bowl.

To make the pizza:
4. Increase the oven temperature to 500°F. Dust a pizza peel with cornmeal (if using a pizza stone), or brush two baking sheets with olive oil.
5. In a medium bowl, toss together the asparagus, olive oil, a squeeze of lemon juice, and the Parmesan. Season with the salt and pepper and toss well.
6. Roll out one of the dough balls to the desired size, and place it on the pizza peel (if using a pizza stone) or on the prepared baking sheet.
7. Spoon half of the ricotta cheese in dollops all over the dough, spreading it evenly. Arrange half of the roasted tomatoes on top, followed by half of the asparagus mixture.
8. Transfer the pizza to the hot pizza stone or oven rack, and bake until the crust is golden and the cheese has melted, 5 to 7 minutes on the pizza stone or 7 to 10 minutes on the baking sheet.
9. Remove the pizza from the oven and transfer it to a cutting board. Let it rest for 5 minutes. Slice and serve.
10. Repeat from step 3 with the remaining dough ball and toppings.

Beef Soup

Prep Time: 10 min **Cook Time:** 40-60 min **Servings:** 4

- 2 teaspoons salt, or more
- 3 carrots, peeled and diced into 2-inch pieces
- 2 celery stalks, cut into 5 to 7 pieces
- 1 large onion, quartered
- Small handful parsley sprigs, stemmed
- 1 cup diced fresh or canned tomatoes
- 2 pounds various cuts of beef

1. Put all the ingredients in a large soup pot. Add enough water to fill the pot to a few inches below the top.
2. Boil the soup for 40 minutes to 1 hour, depending on the cuts of beef used. Tender cuts will take closer to 40 minutes, while tougher cuts will take closer to 1 hour. Skim off any beef fat that rises to the top.
3. Serve this soup as a first course. You can also strain and discard all the non-meat ingredients, chop up the meat, and serve just the broth and the meat.

Nutrition: Calories 465 Cal | Fat 14.3g | Carbs 10 g | Protein 70.1 g | Sodium: 1354 mg

Bread and Pizza

Italian Easter Bread

Prep Time: 20 min
Cook Time: 40 min
Servings: 1 Large Bread

INGREDIENTS

- 1¼ cups whole milk
- 2¼ teaspoons rapid-rise yeast
- Pinch salt
- 5½ tablespoons butter, softened
- 2 eggs, beaten
- ½ cup sugar
- 3½ cups all-purpose flour, plus up to 1 cup more, if needed
- Olive oil, for greasing

DIRECTIONS

1. In a small saucepan over medium-high heat, heat the milk until small bubbles form at the edge. Remove from the heat and transfer the milk into a bowl to cool until lukewarm.
2. In the bowl of a stand mixer, combine the yeast, milk, salt, butter, eggs, and sugar. Using the dough hook attachment, mix until just combined. Add about half the flour and mix until smooth.
3. Slowly add the rest of the flour until a stiff dough forms. Add additional flour, if needed, until the dough is no longer sticky. Knead until smooth.
4. Place the dough in a greased bowl. Cover and let rise in a warm place until the dough has doubled, 45 minutes to 1 hour.
5. Punch the dough down and divide it into three equal pieces. Roll each piece to form a thick rope about 12 inches long. Starting from the top, form a braid.
6. Place the braid on a baking sheet lined with parchment paper.
7. Cover with plastic wrap or a clean kitchen towel and let the dough rise a second time, until doubled, 45 minutes to 1 hour.
8. Preheat the oven to 350ºF and bake until golden, about 40 minutes. Cool on a rack.

Basil Tomato Bread

Prep Time: 15 min
Cook Time: 1 hour and 10 min
Servings: 1 loaf

INGREDIENTS

- 1/2 cup shortening
- 3/4 cup sugar
- 1 large egg
- 2 cups all-purpose flour
- 2-1/2 tsps. baking powder
- 2 tsps. dried basil
- 1 tsp. salt
- 1 cup milk
- 1/2 cup shredded Swiss cheese
- 1/4 cup oil-packed sun-dried tomatoes, chopped

DIRECTIONS

Cream sugar and shortening in a big bowl until fluffy and light; stir in egg well. Mix salt, flour, basil, and baking powder; alternately stir with milk into the creamed mixture. Mix in tomatoes and cheese.
Move to a greased 9-in by 5-in loaf pan. Bake for 50-60mins in a 325 degrees oven until an inserted toothpick in the middle comes out without residue. Cool in the pan for 10mins then move to a wire rack.

NUTRITION: Calories: 178 Calories | Total Carbohydrate: 23 g | Cholesterol: 18 mg | Total Fat: 8 g | Fiber: 1 g | Protein: 4 g | Sodium: 234 mg

Dilly Onion Bread

Prep Time: 10 min
Cook Time: 3 hours
Servings: 1 loaf (16 slices)

- 3/4 cup water (70° to 80°)
- 1 tablespoon butter, softened
- 2 tablespoons sugar
- 3 tablespoons dried minced onion
- 2 tablespoons dried parsley flakes
- 1 tablespoon dill weed
- 1 teaspoon salt
- 1 garlic clove, minced
- 2 cups bread flour
- 1/3 cup whole wheat flour
- 1 tablespoon nonfat dry milk powder
- 2 teaspoons active dry yeast

1. In bread machine pan, put all ingredients following the orders recommended by manufacturer. Choose basic bread setting. Select loaf size, crust color if available. Bake following the directions of bread machine (After 5 mins of mixing, check dough; if needed, put in 1-2 tablespoons water of flour).

NUTRITION: Calories: 77 Cal | Sodium: 159mg | Fiber: 1g | Total Carbohydrate: 16g | Cholesterol: 2mg | Protein: 3g | Total Fat: 1g

Roasted Garlic Bread

Prep Time: 15 min
Cook Time: 35 min
Servings: 8

- 3 heads garlic
- 1/2 cup butter
- 2 tablespoons olive oil
- 1 tablespoon chopped fresh parsley (optional)
- 1 (1 pound) loaf Italian bread
- 2 tablespoons grated Parmesan cheese (optional)

1. Preheat the oven to 350°F (180°C) (175 degrees C). Remove the tops of garlic heads, exposing the tip of each clove. Drizzle olive oil over the garlic on a baking sheet. Bake for 30 minutes, or until garlic is tender.
2. Preheat oven to broil. Place the cut-side up on a baking sheet after slicing the loaf of bread in half horizontally.
3. Squeeze the garlic cloves from their skins into a medium mixing basin. In a large mixing bowl, combine the butter, parsley, and Parmesan cheese until well combined. Spread the mixture on the bread's sliced sides.
4. Toast the bread for around 5 minutes under the broiler.

NUTRITION: Calories: 326 Cal | Carbohydrates: 35.4g | Fat: 17.3g | Protein: 6.9g | Cholesterol: 32mg

Sausage, Potato and Kale Soup

Prep Time: 10 min
Cook Time: 25 min
Servings: 6

- 5 teaspoons olive oil
- 1 (16 ounce) package fettuccini pasta
- 4 shallots, diced
- 3 egg yolks
- 1 large onion, cut into thin strips
- 1/2 cup heavy cream
- 1 pound bacon, cut into strips
- 3/4 cup shredded Parmesan cheese
- 1 clove garlic, chopped
- salt and pepper to taste

1. In a big heavy saucepan, heat the olive oil over medium heat. Soften shallots in a skillet. Cook, stirring frequently, until the bacon is evenly browned. When the bacon is approximately halfway done, add the garlic. Remove the pan from the heat.
2. Boil a large saucepan of lightly salted water. Cook for 8 to 10 minutes, or until pasta is al dente. Return the spaghetti to the saucepan after draining it.
3. Whisk together egg yolks, cream, and shredded Parmesan in a medium mixing basin. Stir in the cream mixture after pouring the bacon mixture over the spaghetti. Salt & pepper to taste.

NUTRITION: Calories 614 | Protein 26 | Fat 28.6g | Cholesterol 166 mg | Sodium 498.1mg | Carbs: 64.8 g

Bread and Pizza

Italian Herb Bread

Prep Time: 30 min | **Cook Time:** 35 min | **Servings:** 24

INGREDIENTS

- 2 (1/4 oz.) packages active dry yeast
- ½ cup grated Romano cheese
- 6 1/2 cups bread flour
- 2 cups water (110 degrees F/45 degrees C)
- 2 tbsp. white sugar
- 4 tbsp. olive oil
- 3 1/2 tsp. salt
- 1 tbsp. dried basil
- 1 tbsp. dried oregano
- 3/4 tsp. garlic powder
- 3/4 tsp. onion powder

1. In a large mixing basin, combine yeast, warm water, and white sugar. Allow it to sit for five minutes or until the mixture has foamed up.
2. In a large mixing bowl, combine the yeast, olive oil, salt, herbs, garlic powder, onion powder, cheese, and 3 cups flour. Mix in the remaining three cups of flour gradually. The dough will be tough.
3. Knead the dough for 5 to 10 minutes, or until smooth and elastic. Place in an oiled basin and turn to coat the dough's surface with oil. Using a damp linen dish towel, cover the dish. Allow one hour for the dough to rise or until it has doubled in size.
4. To get rid of all the air in the dough, punch it down. Make two loaves out of the dough—Bake on a prepared cookie sheet or in two greased 9 x 5-inch loaf pans. Allow rising for 30 minutes or until doubled in size.
5. Preheat oven to 350°F (175°C) and bake for 35 minutes. Remove loaves from pans and cool for at least 15 minutes on wire racks before slicing.

Nutrition: Calories 37 Cal | Fats 3 g | Protein 1.1 g | Cholesterol: 2.6 mg | Sodium: 320.9 g | Carbs: 1.7 g

---

Artichoke Pizza

Prep Time: 15 min | **Cook Time:** 45 min | **Servings:** 2 large pizzas

INGREDIENTS

For the pizza dough:
- 5 cups (1175 ml) all-purpose flour
- 1 ½ teaspoons (7.5 ml) active dry yeast
- 1 teaspoon (5 ml) sea salt
- 2 ¼ (530 ml) cups cold water
- 2 tablespoons (30 ml) extra virgin olive oil

For the toppings:
- 1 cup (235 ml) marinara sauce
- 1 14 oz. (~400 g) (415 ml or similar size) can artichoke hearts
- 1 cup (235 ml) kalamata olives, pitted, chopped
- 1 cup (235 ml) button mushrooms, sliced
- 2 1/3 cups (570 ml) cherry tomatoes, quartered
- 2 tablespoons (30 ml) grated vegan parmesan cheese

DIRECTIONS

1. Program your oven to its highest setting and allow it to heat for 1 hour.
2. Add the flour, sea salt, and yeast into a stand mixer outfitted with the paddle attachment and mix on low speed to combine the ingredients.
3. Add the cold water and a tablespoon (15 ml) of olive oil and mix to combine, then remove the paddle attachment and fasten the dough hook attachment to the machine.
4. Mix the dough for 7-10 minutes on low speed until the pizza dough pulls away from the sides of the stand mixer's bowl and the pizza dough is smooth but slightly sticky.
5. Divide the pizza dough into 6 even portions, then place them into 6 separate greased bowls, cover each pizza dough with plastic wrap and allow them to sit for 1½-2 hours in a warm area.
6. Turn one of the risen pizza doughs onto a floured surface and press or roll out each pizza dough into a circle that is ¼ inch (6 mm) in thickness and 8 to 10 inches (20 to 25 cm) in diameter.
7. Place the pizza dough onto a cookie sheet dusted with cornmeal and continue rolling out the remaining pizza dough.
8. Add 3 tablespoons (45 ml) of marinara sauce to the middle of each pizza, then top with the artichokes, olives, mushrooms, tomatoes, and a sprinkle of vegan parmesan cheese.
9. Bake the pizzas for 7-10 minutes until golden brown around the edges.
10. Serve and enjoy!

Trenton Tomato Pie Pizza

Prep Time: 20 min
Cook Time: 20 min
Servings: makes one 14" diameter pizza

INGREDIENTS

- 1 (28-oz.) can whole peeled tomatoes (preferably San Marzano)
- 3/4 tsp. kosher salt
- 8 oz. Food Processor Pizza Dough or prepared pizza dough, room temperature
- All-purpose flour (for surface)
- 5 oz. part-skim milk mozzarella, shredded (about 1 1/2 cups), divided
- 3/4 tsp. extra-virgin olive oil
- Crushed red pepper flakes (for serving; optional)
- A pizza stone or 2 stackable rimmed baking sheets

DIRECTIONS

1. Put the rack in the bottommost part of the oven. Put a two inverted and stacked baking sheets or a pizza stone on the rack then preheat the oven for at least an hour to 500 degrees
2. In a colander, drain the tomatoes then use your hands to crumble into small pieces; drain again. Move to a medium bowl then mix in salt; set the tomatoes aside.
3. On a lightly floured parchment paper, roll the dough out to a 14-in circle. It should be evenly thin from the middle to the edge. Use plastic wrap to cover the dough if it pulls back when rolling then wait for 5mins.
4. Move the parchment paper with the dough on an inverted baking sheet, big cutting board, or a pizza wheel. Spread 1 1/4 cup cheese then the tomatoes on top. Scatter the remaining quarter cup cheese.
5. Slide the pizza from the parchment carefully on the hot baking stone. Bake for 10-12mins until the crust is deep golden brown.
6. Move to a cutting board then cool the pizza for 2mins; dribble with oil. Slice the pizza into wedges then serve with red pepper flakes, if desired.

Nutrition: Calories: 2540 | Carbohydrate: 287 g | Cholesterol: 196 mg | Fat: 106 g | Protein: 112 g | Sodium: 5377 mg

---

Italian Garlic Bread

Prep Time: 10 min
Cook Time: 6 min
Servings: 8

INGREDIENTS

- 1 tablespoon fresh parsley
- 8 oz Cheddar cheese
- 3 tablespoon basil oil
- 1 teaspoon chili flakes
- 3 oz garlic cloves
- 14 oz white bread
- 1 tablespoon fresh dill
- 4 tablespoon butter

DIRECTIONS

1. Slice the bread roughly.
2. Then preheat the oven to 365 F.
3. Put the sliced bread on the tray and put it in the oven.
4. Bake the bread for 3 minutes on the each side or till the bread gets golden brown color.
5. Meanwhile, place the butter in the blender.
6. Add fresh dill and fresh parsley.
7. After this, add basil oil.
8. Peel the garlic and slice it.
9. Add the sliced garlic to the butter mixture and blend it.
10. Slice Cheddar cheese.
11. When the bread is cooked – remove it from the oven.
12. Spread the bread slices with the blended butter mixture from the both sides.
13. After this, let the bread slices chill little.
14. Put the cheese slices on the bread and serve it immediately.

NUTRITION: Calories: 283 Calories | Fat: 14.4 g | Carbohydrate: 29 g | Fiber: 5 g | Protein: 10 g

Bread and Pizza

Carrot Pizza With Fontina And Red Onion

Prep Time: 35 min
Cook Time: 20 min
Servings: 4 (2 pizzas)

- 2 tbsps. olive oil
- 1/2 medium onion, chopped
- 1/2 lb. carrots (about 3-4 medium carrots), peeled and thinly sliced
- 1/2 cup white wine
- 1/2 tsp. kosher salt
- 1/4 cup mascarpone
- 1/8 tsp. cayenne pepper
- 1/2 lb. prepared pizza dough, room temperature
- All-purpose flour (for surface)
- Olive oil (for brushing)
- 8 oz. Fontina cheese, grated (about 2 cups)
- 1/2 medium red onion, root intact and thinly sliced lengthwise into wedges
- 1 cup (loosely packed) carrot fronds or baby arugula

1. Prepare the carrot puree. On medium-high heat, heat oil in a big pan until it shimmers. Put onions; cook while mixing regularly for 2mins until translucent. Put in carrots; cook while mixing from time to time for 5mins until it starts to brown. Pour in wine; cook while mixing regularly for 2mins until it reduces by 1/2.
2. Turn to medium-low heat, mix in a cup of water and salt until blended; cover. Let it simmer for 15mins until most of the liquid evaporates and the carrots are tender.
3. Move the mixture to a blender; put in a quarter cup water, cayenne, and mascarpone. Take out the stopper on the lid or keep the lid slightly open. Use a towel to cover to avoid splattering hot liquid; puree the mixture until smooth.
4. Prepare the pizza. Put two upturned rimmed baking sheets on the top and bottom thirds of the oven then preheat to 450 degrees F.
5. On a lightly floured surface, halve the dough then shape into two balls. Roll each ball into 6x10-in ovals that can hit the baking sheets. Take the preheated sheets out of the oven then slather oil on the bottoms. Put the dough carefully on the sheets then slather with additional oil. Bake for 5mins until the dough starts to brown.
6. Evenly slather the reserved carrot puree on the pizzas then top with onion and cheese. Bake for 10-12mins until the cheese is bubbling and melted, turn the sheets and swap the places on the racks halfway through baking. Move pizzas on cutting boards; add carrot fronds on top then slice.
7. The carrot puree can be prepared up to two days ahead; chill until ready to make the pizza.

Nutrition: Calories 605 Cal | Fats 38 g | Sodium: 967 mg | Protein 24 g | Fiber: 3 g | Carbs: 40 g

---

Herb Bread

Prep Time: 15 min
Cook Time: 1 hour approx
Servings: 12

- 1/4 cup warm water (110 degrees F/45 degrees C)
- 2 tablespoons margarine
- 3/4 cup milk
- 1 egg
- 1 teaspoon dried parsley
- 1 1/2 teaspoons salt
- 1/2 teaspoon ground nutmeg
- 1 teaspoon rubbed sage
- 2 teaspoons celery seed
- 3 cups bread flour
- 2 tablespoons white sugar
- 1 teaspoon active dry yeast

1. In the pan of bread machine, put ingredients following the order of the manufacturer's suggestions.

Nutrition: Calories: 164 Calories | Total Carbohydrate: 28.1 | Cholesterol: 17 | Protein: 5.4 | Total Fat: 3.2 | Sodium: 325

Eggplant, Tomato, And Fontina Pizza

Prep Time: 45 min
Cook Time: 1 hour and 15 min
Servings: 2 10 inch pizza

INGREDIENTS

- 1 (1 1/2-lb.) eggplant, cut crosswise into 1/4-inch-thick slices
- 1 3/4 tsps. salt
- 3/4 cup packed fresh basil leaves
- 1/4 cup packed fresh mint leaves
- 2 garlic cloves
- 10 oz. grape tomatoes (2 cups), quartered
- 5 tbsps. extra-virgin olive oil plus additional for brushing dough
- Pizza dough
- Flour for dredging
- 1/4 lb. Italian Fontina, rind discarded and cheese cut into 1/4-inch dice (1 cup)
- a pizza stone; parchment paper; a baking peel or rimless baking sheet

DIRECTIONS

1. Prepare the pizza toppings. In a colander, sprinkle 1 1/2 tsp salt on the eggplant; drain in the sink for half an hour while turning the eggplants from time to time.
2. Chop the garlic, mint, and basil together finely; mix with tomatoes in a bowl. Put in a sieve set on top of a bowl to drain.
3. Preheat the broiler.
4. Rinse then pat the eggplant dry in batches between paper towels; firmly press to get rid of the excess moisture. Brush around of 4 tbsp. oil on both side of the slices then cut small stacks; slice the stack into quarters. On two shallow heavy baking pans, put the eggplant pieces in one layer; broil one pan at a time for 7-8mins, around five to six inches from heat until golden brown. Turn the eggplants one time. Bring the eggplant to cool at room temperature.
5. Place the pizza stone on the lower third of the oven then preheat to 500 degrees F. Heat the stone for an hour.
6. Make the pizzas. Don't punch the dough down. Dredge one dough piece gently in flour until coated then move to a parchment paper sheet placed on a baking sheet or baking peel. Hold one edge of the floured dough using both your hands in the air then allow the bottom to touch the parchment paper. Move your hands carefully around the edges of the dough like turning a steering wheel. Let the dough weight stretch the dough roughly to a round of 10-in diameter. Place the round on the parchment then adjust the shape as necessary.
7. Get rid of all the exuded liquid from tomatoes. In a bowl, mix tomatoes, the remaining a quarter tsp. salt, and remaining tbsp. oil. Brush oil on the dough round then sprinkle 1/2 of tomatoes, 1/2 of cheese, and 1/2 of cheese on top, keep an inch of border around the edge. Line the far edge of the peel with the far edge of the pizza stone; tilt the peel down then gently jerk to begin moving the pizza. Slide the pizza and parchment onto the stone; bake for 12-15mins until the cheese is bubbling and the crust is golden brown. Take the pizza out of the oven by sliding the peel beneath the paper. Move to a cutting board then get rid of the parchment paper.
8. As you bake the first pizza, prepare the second one on another parchment sheet. Bake in the same way.

NUTRITION: Calories: 2529 | Total Carbohydrate: 386 g | Cholesterol: 97 mg | Total Fat: 66 g | Fiber: 32 g | Protein: 94 g | Sodium: 4977 mg | Saturated Fat: 26 g

Quick Italian Vegetable Soup

Prep Time 15 min | **Cook Time** 30 min | **Servings** 6

INGREDIENTS

- 1 tablespoon olive oil
- 1 medium onion, chopped
- 2 thin strips carrots, sliced
- 2 stalks celery, sliced
- 1 (16 ounce) can diced plum tomatoes
- 2 teaspoons Italian seasoning
- 2 cubes beef bouillon
- 6 cups water
- 2 medium (blank)s zucchinis, quartered and sliced
- 2 cups sliced cabbage
- 1 teaspoon garlic salt
- 1 teaspoon salt and ground black pepper to taste
- ½ cup freshly grated Parmesan cheese

DIRECTIONS

1. In a large stockpot, heat the oil over medium-high heat. For 5-7 minutes, sauté onion, carrot, and celery until onion is transparent and vegetables are soft. Cook for another 5 minutes, stirring often, after adding the tomatoes and Italian spice.
2. In a small bowl, dissolve the bouillon cubes in water and stir them into the vegetables. Reduce the heat and simmer for about 10 minutes. Add the zucchini and cabbage, season with garlic salt, and simmer for another 5 minutes, or until soft. Season with salt and pepper, then serve.

NUTRITION: Calories 93 Cal | Protein 4.9g | Carbohydrates 10g | Fat 4.5g | Cholesterol 5.9mg | Sodium 1210.2mg |

Basic Focaccia with Basil

Prep Time 15 min | **Cook Time** 25 min | **Servings** 1 Large Focaccia

INGREDIENTS

- 1 packet rapid-rise yeast
- 1 teaspoon sugar
- 1½ cups warm water, divided
- 3 tablespoons olive oil, plus more for greasing, divided
- 5 to 6 cups all-purpose flour, divided
- 2 teaspoons salt
- Extra-virgin olive oil, for drizzling
- ½ cup basil leaves, finely chopped

DIRECTIONS

1. In the mixing bowl of a stand mixer, combine the yeast, sugar, and ½ cup of warm water. Let stand for several minutes.
2. Add the remaining 1 cup of warm water, 3 tablespoons of oil, 5 cups of flour, and the salt. Using the dough hook attachment, mix the dough on low speed for 5 to 6 minutes. If the dough is sticky, add more flour as needed, up to 1 additional cup.
3. Transfer the dough to a large oiled bowl. Cover with plastic wrap and allow to double in size, 1 to 2 hours.
4. Punch the dough down and generously oil a baking sheet. Add the dough to the baking sheet and spread it to the edge of the pan. Loosely cover and allow 30 to 40 minutes for a second rise. Preheat the oven to 400°F.
5. Indent the dough all over the top with your thumbs, drizzle with oil, and bake for 20 minutes. Remove from the oven, drizzle with extra-virgin olive oil, and sprinkle with the basil. Bake for an additional 5 to 7 minutes.

Ciabatta Bread

Prep Time: 4 hour and 10 min
Cook Time: 25 min
Servings: 8

INGREDIENTS

- *For the ciabatta starter:*
- 1/8 teaspoon (0.6 ml) active dry yeast
- 2 tablespoons (30 ml) warm water
- ½ cup (120 ml) whole wheat flour
- ½ cup (120 ml) bread flour
- 1/3 cup (80 ml) distilled room temperature water
- *For the ciabatta bread:*
- 1 ½ cups+1 tablespoon (375 ml) warm water
- ½ teaspoon (2.5 ml) active dry yeast
- 2 cups (470 ml) bread flour
- ½ teaspoon (2.5 ml) fine sea salt
- 1 tablespoon (15 ml) extra-virgin olive oil

DIRECTIONS

1. To make the starter, combine the yeast with two tablespoons (30 ml) of water in a bowl and let it bloom for 5 minutes.
2. Add the whole wheat and bread flour, and water and mix until combined.
3. Cover the starter with plastic wrap and let sit at room temperature for 12 hours or overnight.
4. To make the ciabatta bread, place the yeast and two tablespoons (30 ml) of water into a stand mixer's bowl fitted with the dough hook and allow to sit for 5 minutes.
5. Add the remaining water, bread flour, salt, and olive oil, and mix until a shaggy dough forms. Knead the dough for 5-6 minutes, then place it into a bowl greased with oil, cover the ciabatta dough with plastic wrap and let rise for 1 ½ to 2 hours or until doubled in volume.
6. Transfer the ciabatta dough to a floured surface and divide it into portions. Shape each ciabatta dough into a loaf and place them on a parchment-lined cookie sheet.
7. Cut a singular slit down the length of each ciabatta loaf with a sharp knife or sourdough lame, then cover the loaves with a clean damp kitchen towel and let rise for 1 ½ to 2 hours or until doubled in volume.
8. Program the oven to 400° F (205° C) during the last 30 minutes of the ciabatta's rising time.
9. Spray the ciabatta loaves lightly with water and bake the ciabatta bread for 20-25 minutes until golden.
10. Place the ciabatta bread onto a wire rack to cool completely before slicing.
11. Serve and enjoy!

Roman "Egg Drop" Soup

Prep Time: 15 min
Cook Time: 20 min
Servings: 6

INGREDIENTS

- 1/3 cup freshly grated Grana Padano, plus more for serving
- 1¼ teaspoons kosher salt
- 4 big eggs
- 4 cups packed spinach leaves, shredded
- 8 cups defatted homemade Chicken Stock
- Freshly ground black pepper

DIRECTIONS

1. In a moderate-sized pot, bring the stock to a simmer. Once it is simmering, put in 1 teaspoon salt and the spinach and cook until soft, approximately three minutes.
2. In the meantime, in a moderate-sized bowl, whisk together eggs, grated cheese, rest of the ¼ teaspoon salt, and some freshly ground black pepper to taste.
3. Once the spinach is soft, put in about a third of the egg mixture to the soup, while constantly whisking the soup where the egg is falling, to make shreds of the eggs. Put in and whisk rest of the eggs in two more batches, allowing the soup to return to its boiling point between additions. Once all of the eggs have been added, bring soup to a final boil, and use the whisk to break up any big clusters of eggs. Serve soup with additional grated cheese.

Bread and Pizza

Crusty Hoagie Bread

Prep Time: 1 hour and 10 min
Cook Time: 25 min
Servings: 8

INGREDIENTS
- 1 to 1 ¼ cups (235-295 ml) warm water
- 2 tablespoons (30 ml) honey
- 2 ¼ teaspoons (33 ml) active dry yeast
- 4 cups (960 ml) bread flour
- ½ cup (120 ml) warm almond milk
- 1 teaspoon (5 ml) sea salt
- ¼ cup (56.5 g/60 ml) cold butter, cubed

DIRECTIONS
1. Combine ¼ cup (60 ml) warm water, the honey, and active dry yeast in a stand mixer's bowl and allow the yeast mixture to bloom for 5-10 minutes.
2. Fasten the dough hook to the machine, and add the remaining water, 2 cups (470 ml) of flour, and the almond milk and mix on low until combined.
3. Add the salt and the remaining bread flour, increase the mixer's speed, and mix until a dough forms.
4. Add the cold butter cubes one a time and mix until the butter cubes blend into the dough and the dough pulls away from the bowl's sides.
5. Place the dough into a bowl greased with oil, cover with plastic wrap, and let the dough sit for 1 hour or until doubled in size.
6. Punch the dough down, place it onto a lightly floured surface, and divide it into eight even portions.
7. Shape the dough into eight small loaves and place them onto a parchment-lined cookie sheet. Cover the hoagie bread with a clean damp kitchen towel and allow them to rise for 30 minutes.
8. Program your oven to 375° F (190° C) during the last 15 minutes of rising time.
9. Bake the hoagie rolls for 23-25 minutes or until golden, then place them on a wire rack to cool completely.
10. Serve and enjoy!

Bell Pasta Soup

Prep Time: 10 min
Cook Time: 20 min
Servings: 8

INGREDIENTS
- 1 tbsp olive oil
- 1 onion, chopped
- 2 cloves garlic, minced
- 1 red bell pepper, chopped
- 3 C. low fat, low chicken broth
- 1 C. canned whole tomatoes, chopped
- 1 1/2 C. kidney beans, cooked
- 2 tsps chopped fresh thyme
- 1/2 C. chopped spinach
- 1 C. seashell pasta
- ground black pepper to taste

DIRECTIONS
1. Place a large pot on medium heat. Heat the oil in it. Add the onion and garlic then cook them for 5 min. Stir in the bell pepper and cook them for 3 min.
2. Stir in the broth, tomatoes and beans. Cook them until they start boiling. Lower the heat and simmer the soup for 20 min.
3. Add the thyme, spinach and pasta. Cook the soup for 5 min. Adjust the seasoning of the soup. Serve it warm. Enjoy.

NUTRITION: Calories 174 kcal | Fat:3.1 g | Carbohydrates:29g | Protein 8 g | Cholesterol: 0 mg | Sodium :409 mg

Smokey Mediter- Soup

Prep Time: 10 min
Cook Time: 40 min
Servings: 4

INGREDIENTS

- 1 garlic clove, minced
- 2 garlic cloves, sliced
- 2 teaspoons thyme, chopped
- 1 egg, whisked
- 12 ounces pork meat, ground
- 12 ounces veal, ground
- Salt and black pepper to the taste
- 3 ounces manchego, grated
- A pinch of saffron
- 15 ounces canned tomatoes, crushed
- 2 tablespoons extra virgin olive oil
- 1/3 cup panko
- 4 cups chicken stock
- 1 tablespoons parsley, chopped
- 8 ounces pasta

DIRECTIONS

1. In a bowl, mix veal with pork, 1 garlic clove, 1 teaspoon thyme, ¼ teaspoon paprika, salt, pepper to the taste, egg, manchego a panko and stir very well.
2. Shape 20 meatballs from this mix using your wet hands and put them on a plate.
3. Heat up a pan with 1 and ½ tablespoons oil over medium high heat, add half of the meatballs, cook for 2 minutes on each side, transfer to paper towels, drain grease and put on a plate.
4. Repeat this with the rest of the meatballs.
5. Heat up the pot with the rest of the oil, add sliced garlic, stir and cook for 1 minute.
6. Add the rest of the thyme, the rest of the paprika, saffron, stock and tomatoes, stir and cook for 2 minutes.
7. Add meatballs, stir, reduce heat to medium low, cook for 25 minutes and season with salt and pepper.
8. Cook pasta is accruing to instructions, drain them, put into a bowl and mix with ½ cup soup.
9. Divide pasta into soup bowls, add soup and meatballs on top, sprinkle parsley all over and serve.

Nutrition: Calories 380 Cal | Fat 17g | Fiber 2g | Carbohydrates 28g | Protein 26g

Italian Halibut Chowder

Prep Time: 20 min
Cook Time: 1 hour and 10 min
Servings: 8

INGREDIENTS

- 2 1/4 lb. cubed halibut steaks
- 1 red bell pepper, chopped
- 1 onion, chopped
- 3 stalks celery, chopped
- 3 cloves garlic, minced
- ¼ cup olive oil
- 1 cup tomato juice
- ½ cup apple juice
- 2 16oz. cans whole peeled tomatoes, mashed
- 2 tbsp. chopped fresh parsley
- ½ teaspoon salt
- ½ teaspoon dried basil
- ⅛ teaspoon dried thyme
- A pinch of freshly ground black pepper

DIRECTIONS

1. In a skillet, cook the peppers, celery, onion, and garlic until soft. Combine the tomato juice or water, apple juice, mashed tomatoes, and herbs in a large mixing bowl—Cook for 30 minutes on low heat.
2. Toss the halibut pieces into the soup. Cook for 30 minutes or until the halibut is done. Season with salt and pepper to taste.

NUTRITION: Calories: 263 | Calories | Total Fat: 10.3 g | Sodium: 399.7 g | Carbs: 10.7 g | Cholesterol: 17 | Protein: 31.2 g

Bread and Pizza

Vegetables

Zucchini Pesto

Prep Time: 10 min | **Cook Time:** 25 min | **Servings:** 4

INGREDIENTS
- 1/4 cup fresh basil
- 1 clove garlic (or more to taste)
- 3 medium zucchini, chunked and steamed (reserve liquid)
- 1 to 2 tablespoons olive oil
- 1 cup low-fat ricotta cheese
- Salt and pepper to taste
- 1 tablespoon Parmesan cheese, grated

DIRECTIONS
1. Place basil and garlic into a blender or food processor and process until finely chopped. Add remaining ingredients and puree until smooth.
2. Adjust seasoning; and add reserved zucchini liquid if sauce is too thick (chicken stock may also be used - it will give a richer flavor). Toss with warm pasta, preferably angel hair or thin spaghetti.

Horseradish Mashed Potatoes Side Dish

Prep Time: 20 min | **Cook Time:** 40 min | **Servings:** 6

INGREDIENTS
- 1 cup half-and-half
- 1 cup milk
- 1 stick unsalted butter
- 2 teaspoons kosher salt
- 2-inch piece fresh horseradish root, peeled and grated (about ½ cup)
- 3 pounds russet potatoes, all about the same size

DIRECTIONS
1. Put the unpeeled whole potatoes in a big pot with cold water to cover by about 2 inches. Heat to a simmer, and cook until soft, approximately thirty to forty minutes. Drain, and allow it to sit until just sufficiently cool to peel.
2. While the potatoes cool, mix the butter, half-and-half, milk, and salt in the cooking pot using low heat, just until the butter melts.
3. Use a ricer, and press the still-warm potatoes through into the butter mixture. Put in the horseradish, and stir until the desired smoothness is achieved. Adjust seasoning, and serve instantly.

Zesty Zucchini

Prep Time: 10 min | **Cook Time:** 0 min | **Servings:** 4

INGREDIENTS
- 1/3 cup vegetable oil
- 1/4 cup white wine vinegar
- 1 tablespoon minced fresh basil or 1 teaspoon dried basil
- 1/2 teaspoon salt
- 1/4 teaspoon pepper
- 1/4 teaspoon garlic powder
- 2 to 3 medium zucchini, sliced

DIRECTIONS
1. Beat the first 6 ingredients together in a large bowl. Put in zucchini and toss. Cool in the fridge, then serve.

Nutrition: Calories: 180 | Total Carbs: 4 g | Cholesterol: 0 mg | Total Fat: 18 g | Protein: 1 g | Sodium: 298 mg | Fiber: 1 g

Green Bean in Bread Crumbs

Prep Time 15 min **Cook Time** 10 min **Servings** 4

- 1 pound fresh green beans, washed and trimmed
- 1/4 teaspoon garlic powder
- 1/2 cup water
- 1/4 teaspoon dried oregano
- 1/4 cup Italian-style seasoned bread crumbs
- 1/4 teaspoon dried basil
- 1/4 cup olive oil
- 1/4 cup grated Parmesan cheese
- salt and pepper to taste

1. In a medium pot, combine green beans and 1/2 cup water. Bring to a boil, covered. Reduce heat to medium and simmer for 10 minutes, or until beans are tender. Drain thoroughly.
2. Toss beans with bread crumbs, olive oil, salt, pepper, garlic powder, oregano, and basil in a medium serving bowl. Toss the beans in the mixture until they are evenly covered. Serve with a sprinkling of Parmesan cheese.

Nutrition: Calories: 210 | Carbohydrates: 13.6g | Fat: 15.8g | Protein: 5.5g | Cholesterol: 6mg

Italian Garlic Mushrooms

Prep Time 15 min **Cook Time** 25 min **Servings** 8

- 1 tsp. ground black pepper
- 4 oz. cheddar cheese
- 2 tbsp. minced garlic
- 1 tbsp. Italian seasoning
- 1 tbsp. green chives
- 1 lb. mushroom
- ¼ tsp. salt
- 1 tsp. olive oil

1. Slice the mushrooms and sprinkle them with salt.
2. Combine the minced garlic with the ground black pepper and olive oil.
3. Then toss the minced garlic mixture in the pan and roast it for 1 minute.
4. After this, add sliced mushrooms.
5. Simmer the mixture for 15 minutes. Stir it constantly. You should not get the brown color of the ingredients.
6. Then sprinkle the dish with Italian seasoning and chives.
7. Grate cheddar cheese.
8. Then add the grated cheese and mix the dish carefully until the cheese is melted.
9. Place the cooked meal on the serving plates and serve the dish hot.

Balsamic Roasted Vegetables

Prep Time 10 min **Cook Time** 00 min **Servings** 6

- 1 large zucchini, cut into ½-inch (1.25 cm) rounds diagonally
- 2 summer squash, cut into ½-inch (1.25 cm) rounds diagonally
- 8 oz. (226 g) (1 cup/235 ml) button mushrooms, sliced
- 1 head cauliflower, sliced into florets
- 1 large eggplant cup into ½-inch (1.25 cm) rounds
- 2 tablespoons (30 ml) olive oil
- 2 tablespoons (30 ml) balsamic vinegar
- 1 tablespoon (15 ml) Italian seasoning
- 1 teaspoon (5 ml) garlic powder
- 1 teaspoon (5 ml) sea salt
- ½ teaspoon (2.5 ml) black pepper.

1. Program your oven to 450° F (230° C).
2. Place the zucchini, summer squash, mushrooms, cauliflower, eggplant, olive oil, balsamic vinegar, Italian seasoning, sea salt, and pepper into a bowl and toss to combine.
3. Spread the vegetable medley onto a non-stick cookie sheet in an even layer and roast them for 10 minutes.
4. Turn the roasted vegetables over and cook them for an additional 10 minutes until tender.
5. Serve and enjoy!

Vegetables

Vegetarian Strata

Prep Time 20 min   **Cook Time** 25 min   **Servings** 12

INGREDIENTS

- 2 tsp. minced fresh thyme or 1/2 tsp. dried thyme
- 1 medium zucchini
- 6 eggs, lightly beaten
- 2 cups fat-free milk
- 1 medium red onion
- 1-3/4 cups Parmesan cheese
- 1/4 tsp. ground nutmeg
- 1 medium sweet red pepper, finely chopped
- 2 tsp. olive oil
- 3 garlic cloves, minced
- 1/2 tsp. salt
- 1 loaf (1 lb.) day-old French bread
- 2 packages (5.3-oz each) fresh goat cheese
- 1/4 tsp. pepper
- 1 cup sliced baby portobello mushrooms

DIRECTIONS

1. Sauté onion, mushrooms, red pepper, and zucchini in oil in a large skillet until they become tender. Put in pepper, salt, thyme, and garlic; sauté for 1 more minute.
2. In a greased 13x9-inch baking dish, arrange Parmesan cheese, goat cheese, zucchini mixture, and 1/2 bread cubes in a layer in reverse order. Repeat the process.
3. Beat together nutmeg, milk, and eggs in a small bowl. Place the blend over the top. Put in the fridge, covered, overnight.
4. Before baking, take it out from the fridge for half an hour. Set an oven to 350 degrees and start preheating. Uncover and bake until a knife comes out clean after inserted in the center, or for 45-50 minutes. Before cutting, allow standing for 10 minutes.

Eggplant Parmesan

Prep Time 25 min   **Cook Time** 45 min   **Servings** 8

INGREDIENTS

- 1 eggplant, sliced
- 1/2 cup grated Parmesan cheese
- 1 1/2 tablespoons salt
- 1 egg, beaten
- 8 tablespoons olive oil
- 1/2 cup chopped fresh basil
- 8 ounces ricotta cheese
- 4 cups pasta sauce
- 6 ounces shredded mozzarella cheese

DIRECTIONS

1. Using a 34-inch slicer, cut the eggplant into 34-inch slices. Season the eggplant slices on both sides with salt. Place the slices in a sieve with a dish underneath to catch the liquid that will evaporate as the eggplant sweats. Allow for 30 minutes of resting time.
2. Preheat the oven to 350 degrees Fahrenheit (175 degrees C). Combine the ricotta, mozzarella, and 1/4 cup Parmesan cheese in a medium mixing basin. Combine the egg and basil in a mixing bowl.
3. Rinse the eggplant in cool water until it is completely free of salt. Heat 4 tbsp. olive oil in large skillet over medium heat. Brown each side of one layer of eggplant in the pan. Repeat with the remaining eggplant pieces, adding more oil as needed.
4. 1 1/2 cups spaghetti sauce, evenly spread in a 9x13 inch baking dish On top of the sauce, arrange a single layer of eggplant slices. 1/2 of the cheese mixture should be placed on top of the eggplant. Continue layering until all of the eggplant and cheese mixture has been used. Pour the remaining sauce over the layers, then top with the remaining Parmesan cheese.
5. Bake for about 45 minutes, or until sauce is bubbling, in a preheated oven.

Broccoli Flan with Anchovy Sauce

Prep Time 30 min **Cook Time** 40 min **Servings** 4

INGREDIENTS

- 9 oz. (250 g) broccoli, or about 1 1/2 cups florets 2/3 mug (150 ml) lotion.
- 1 oz. (25 g) grated Parmigiano-Reggiano cheese, or concerning 1/4 mug 3 big eggs.
- 2 tsp. (10 g) unsalted butter Salt and pepper.

FOR Sauce
- 2 salted anchovies.
- 2 tablespoon. (30 ml) extra-virgin olive oil.

DIRECTIONS

1. Warm oven to 300 ° F (150 ° C). steam a medium pot of salted water. Add broc -coli and also cook until stems hurt when pierced with a fork. Dive in ice water, after that drain.
2. Put broccoli in a blender or food processor. Include cream, Parmigiano-Reggiano cheese, and also eggs. Mix up until smooth. Season with Salt and pepper butter individual ramekins or timbale mold and mildews as well as full of broccoli blend. Put ramekins in a warm water bathroom (a bain-marie or a toasting frying pan filled with warm water midway up sides of ramekins) and also cook For around 40 minutes
3. Meanwhile, prepare anchovy Sauce Wash anchovies, fillet them if necessary, placed them in mixer with oil as well as blend until smooth.
4. When flans are prepared, eliminate them from water bathroom as well as let them trendy slightly. Invert flans onto specific serving plates and also garnish with anchovy Sauce

---

Spinach Manicotti with Italian Sausage

Prep Time 15 min **Cook Time** 1 hour and 15 min **Servings** 6

INGREDIENTS

- 250 grams fresh spinach
- 1 lb. bulk Italian sausage
- 1 carton (24oz.) small curd cottage cheese
- 1 package (12oz.)shredded mozzarella cheese, divided
- 12 piece (blank)s manicotti shells
- 2 jars (24oz.) jars spaghetti sauce

DIRECTIONS

1. Preheat the oven to 350 degrees Fahrenheit (175 degrees C).
2. Bring a pot of water to a boil, then submerge spinach in the boiling water for 2 minutes, or until dark green and softened. Excess moisture should be drained and squeezed out.
3. Cook sausage in a pan over medium heat, tossing frequently, until browned and crumbled, about 10 minutes. Remove any excess grease. In a mixing dish, combine the spinach and sausage. Stir up the cottage cheese and 8 ounces of mozzarella cheese with the sausage and spinach until everything is well mixed.
4. Stuff uncooked manicotti shells with stuffing using your fingers. Place stuffed manicotti side by side in a baking tray and pour both jars of sauce over them.
5. Bake in the preheated oven until manicotti are tender but still slightly firm to the bite and the filling is hot, from 1-1.25 hours. Serve by sprinkling the remaining 4 ounces of mozzarella cheese over the dish and allowing it to melt.

NUTRITION: Calories: 764.7 Cal | Carbs: 63.5 g | Fat: 35.4 g | Protein: 47.6 g | Cholesterol: 87.6 mg | Sodium 2394.7mg

Vegetables

Turnip Greens and Pancetta

Prep Time: 15 min
Cook Time: 20 min
Servings: 6

INGREDIENTS

- ¼ cup extra-virgin olive oil
- ½ teaspoon crushed red pepper flakes
- 1 big onion, cut
- 2 teaspoons kosher salt
- 3 pounds turnip greens, trimmed, washed, spun dry, and torn into big chunks
- 6-ounce chunk pancetta, cut into matchsticks

DIRECTIONS

1. In a big Dutch oven, heat the olive oil on moderate heat. Put in the pancetta, and cook until the fat is rendered and the pancetta is almost crisp, approximately 4 minutes.
2. Put in the onion, and cook, stirring once in a while, until it is wilted, approximately five minutes.
3. Put in the greens, and stir to coat them in the oil. Sprinkle with salt and red pepper flakes. Put in ½ cup water, cover, and simmer on moderate heat until the greens are wilted, approximately fifteen minutes.
4. Uncover, adjust heat so the liquid is just simmering, and cook until soft, approximately ten to fifteen minutes more. Serve hot.

Zucchini Crepes

Prep Time: 15 min
Cook Time: 25 min
Servings: 6

INGREDIENTS

- 1 cup all-purpose flour
- 2 large eggs
- 1/2 cup egg substitute
- 1-1/2 cups fat-free milk
- 3/4 tsp. salt

FILLING:

- 1 large onion, chopped
- 1-1/2 cups cheddar cheese
- 1 medium green pepper, chopped
- 1/8 tsp. pepper
- 1 cup sliced fresh mushrooms
- 1 tbsp. canola oil
- 1 medium zucchini, shredded and squeezed dry
- 2 medium tomatoes, chopped and seeded
- 1/4 tsp. salt
- 1/4 tsp. dried oregano
- 1-1/2 cups meatless spaghetti sauce

DIRECTIONS

1. Combine salt, milk, egg substitute, eggs, and flour in a large bowl until smooth. Keep in the refrigerator for 1 hour, covered.
2. Use cooking spray to coat an 8-inch nonstick skillet, then heat; place about 1/4 cup batter into the middle of the skillet. Lift and rotate pan to equally coat bottom. Cook until the top looks dry; flip and cook for 15-20 seconds more. Take to a wire rack. Continue with remaining batter; apply cooking spray to coat as necessary.
3. Once cool, pile crepes with paper towels or waxed paper in between. In a large pan, sauté mushrooms, green pepper, and onion in oil until soft. Stir in zucchini; sauté for 2-3 minutes more. Take off from heat; mix in pepper, oregano, salt, 1 cup of cheese, and tomatoes.
4. Place onto crepes and roll-up. Pour spaghetti sauce over crepes and spread. Preheat the oven to 350°F and bake for 15-20 minutes, covered. Serve.

Italian-Style Baked Zucchini

Prep Time: 25 min **Cook Time:** 50 min **Servings:** 6

INGREDIENTS

- 2 tablespoons butter
- 6 zucchini, cut in 1/4 inch slices and quartered
- 1/3 cup red bell pepper, seeded and chopped
- 1 teaspoon Italian seasoning
- 1/2 teaspoon salt
- 1/4 teaspoon black pepper
- 1/4 teaspoon garlic powder
- 4 eggs
- 1 cup half and half
- 1 cup shredded provolone cheese
- 2 tablespoons flour
- 1/4 cup grated Romano cheese

DIRECTIONS

1. In a large skillet over medium heat, melt butter. Sauté zucchini, bell pepper, Italian seasoning, salt, pepper and garlic powder until vegetables are tender yet crisp.
2. In a large bowl, beat eggs until foamy; stir in cream, provolone cheese and flour. Add vegetable mixture and pour into a well-buttered baking dish. Sprinkle Romano cheese over the top of the mixture. Bake 40 to 45 minutes at 350 degrees F. until a knife inserted into the center comes out clean. Let stand for 5 minutes before serving.

Whole Braised Cauliflower

Prep Time: 15 min **Cook Time:** 30 min **Servings:** 4

INGREDIENTS

- ¼ teaspoon crushed red pepper flakes
- 1 big head cauliflower, cored, but soft leaves left attached (about 2 pounds)
- 1 big onion, cut
- 1 teaspoon kosher salt
- 2 tablespoons extra-virgin olive oil
- 4 ounces thick-cut bacon, cut into ½-inch pieces
- One 28-ounce can Italian plum tomatoes, preferably San Marzano, crushed using your hands

DIRECTIONS

1. In a pot just big enough to hold the cauliflower with a few inches to spare around the edges, heat the olive oil on moderate heat, put in the bacon, and cook until the fat is rendered and the bacon is almost crunchy, approximately 4 minutes. Put in the onion, and cook until it is wilted, approximately
2. Set the cauliflower, bottom side down, on top of the onion. Pour the tomatoes over it, along with 1 cup water sloshed from the tomato can to clean it out. Sprinkle with salt and crushed red pepper flakes. Heat to a simmer, and cover. Simmer until the cauliflower is soft but not falling apart, approximately twenty-five minutes.
3. Take the cauliflower using a spatula to a cutting board, and slice into ½-inch wedges. Serve in a deep bowl with the sauce. Or serve whole with the sauce, and let everyone fish out a portion with a serving spoon.

NUTRITION: Calories: 106 Calories | Fat: 4.8 g | Carbohydrate: 12.3 g | Protein: 4.2 g

Vegetables

Zucchini With Anchovies And Capers

Prep Time 15 min | **Cook Time** 17 min | **Servings** 6

INGREDIENTS
- ¼ cup drained tiny capers in brine
- 1 teaspoon kosher salt
- 2½ pounds small zucchini
- 4 garlic cloves, crushed and peeled
- 6 anchovy fillets, finely chopped
- 6 tablespoons extra-virgin olive oil

DIRECTIONS
1. In the pan of bread machine, put ingredients following the order of the manufacturer's suggestions. Trim the ends of the zucchini, and slice them into ¼-inch-thick sticks, 2 to 3 inches long. Heat the olive oil in a big frying pan on moderate heat. Put in the garlic cloves, cook for one minute or so, until sizzling, then put in the chopped anchovies. Cook while stirring, until the anchovies melt in the oil, approximately 1 to two minutes. Spread the zucchini sticks in the frying pan, and toss and stir to coat them in oil. Sprinkle with salt, and cook, stirring once in a while, until the zucchini is thoroughly cooked, limp, and lightly caramelized, approximately fifteen minutes.
2. Put in the capers, and cook one more minute or two to combine the flavors. Remove garlic and serve hot or at room temperature.

Pan Fried Asparagus

Prep Time 5 min | **Cook Time** 15 min | **Servings** 4

INGREDIENTS
- 1/4 cup butter
- 1/4 teaspoon ground black pepper
- 2 tablespoons olive oil
- 3 cloves garlic, minced
- 1 teaspoon coarse salt
- 1 pound fresh asparagus spears, trimmed

DIRECTIONS
1. In a skillet over medium-high heat, melt the butter.
2. Combine the olive oil, salt, and pepper in a mixing bowl.
3. Cook garlic for a minute in butter, but don't let it brown.
4. Cook for 10 minutes, flipping asparagus halfway through to achieve equal cooking.

Nutrition: Calories: 188 | Carbohydrates: 5.2g | Fat: 18.4g | Protein: 2.8g | Cholesterol: 31mg

Easy Baked Mushrooms

Prep Time 10 min | **Cook Time** 20 min | **Servings** 4

INGREDIENTS
- 1 pound medium fresh mushrooms, halved
- 2 tablespoons olive oil
- 1/4 cup seasoned bread crumbs
- 1/4 teaspoon garlic powder
- 1/4 teaspoon pepper
- Fresh parsley, optional

DIRECTIONS
1. On a baking sheet, add mushroom. Drizzle over with oil and toss to coat well. Mix together pepper, garlic powder and bread crumbs in a small bowl, then sprinkle over mushrooms.
2. Bake at 425° without a cover until browned slightly, about 18 to 20 minutes. Decorate with parsley if wanted.

Nutrition: Calories: 116 cal | Total Carbs: 10 g | Total Fat: 8 g | Protein: 4 g | Sodium: 112 mg | Fiber: 2 g

Stuffed Cabbage

Prep Time: 10 min
Cook Time: 1 hour
Servings: 4

INGREDIENTS

- 1 medium onion, minced
- 3 cloves of garlic, minced
- 6 tablespoons chopped parsley
- 6 Tbs. bread crumbs
- 2 eggs, Salt & Pepper to taste
- 1 cup long grain rice, cooked
- 2 lb. ground beef
- ½ cup grated Pecorino Romano
- 1 medium Head Savoy Cabbage, about 2 lbs.
- ½ cup chicken broth
- ½ stick of Butter
- ¼ cup Olive Oil
- 2 cups tomato sauce

DIRECTIONS

1. Cook rice according to directions on package, then let cool. You will end up with 2 cups rice.
2. Bring a large pot of salted water to the boil. Cut the bottom off of the cabbage. Cut the core out of the cabbage. Cook the cabbage in boiling water for 4-5 minutes, until the cabbage leaves are tender, yet still slightly firm. Drain cabbage and let cool.
3. In a large mixing bowl, add cooled the rice, onion, garlic, parsley, ground beef, and breadcrumbs.
4. Season the beef liberally with slat and pepper. Mix with hands. Add cheese, a ½ a cup of the tomato sauce, and eggs, and mix thoroughly.
5. Take a small handful of the meat mixture and fill each cabbage leave. Place a small amount of the meat mixture about 3 inches from the end of a cabbage leave. Fold the end over the meat. Fold sides in, and then roll cabbage leave up to close. Roll cabbage leaves until all the meat mixture is gone.
6. Heat oven to 400 degrees. Coat a shallow glass or ceramic baking pan with the olive oil. Place half of the remaining tomato sauce into pan. Place all the rolled cabbages neatly into pan. Cover with remaining tomato sauce. Add chicken Broth and dot with butter on top.
7. Cook in oven at 400 degrees for 12 minutes. Lower heat to 350 and continue cooking for about 30 minutes until the meat inside the cabbage is fully cooked.
8. Take out of oven and let rest for 10 minutes before serving. Serve each person 3 or 4 Stuffed Cabbages with a little sauce. You may serve with roast, boiled, or mashed potatoes or whatever you like.

Cool Cucumber Pasta

Prep Time: 20 min
Cook Time: 20 min
Servings: 8

INGREDIENTS

- 8 oz. uncooked penne pasta
- 1 tbsp. canola oil
- 2 medium cucumbers, thinly sliced
- 1 medium onion, thinly sliced
- 1-1/2 cups sugar
- 1 cup water
- 3/4 cup white vinegar
- 1 tbsp. prepared mustard
- 1 tbsp. dried parsley flakes
- 1 tsp. salt
- 1 tsp. pepper
- 1/2 tsp. garlic salt

DIRECTIONS

1. Cook pasta according to package directions; drain and rinse with cool water. Combine the cooked pasta, onion, cucumbers, and oil in a large mixing basin.
2. In a small mixing dish, combine the remaining ingredients. Add to the salad and toss to incorporate.
3. Cover and chill for 4 hours, tossing occasionally. To eat, use a slotted spoon.
4. Place any leftovers in the refrigerator.

NUTRITION: Calories: 226 Calories | Total Carbs: 50 g | Cholesterol: 0 mg | Total Fat: 2 g | Fiber: 2 g | Protein: 4 g | Sodium: 346 mg

Vegetables

Roast Tuscan Potatoes

Prep Time: 25 min
Cook Time: 40 min
Servings: 4

INGREDIENTS
- 5 Idaho Baking Potatoes
- ¼ cup Olive Oil
- ¼ teaspoon each of Sea Salt & Black Pepper
- 3 sprigs fresh Rosemary
- 5 cloves of Garlic, peeled and left whole

DIRECTIONS
1. Wash the potatoes and cut in half long-ways. Then cut each half-potato in-half length-ways again, then cut each of these long strips into 5 pieces each. Cut each potato this way (you want cubes 1/2 to 2" each).
2. Place all the ingredients except the garlic in a glass or ceramic baking dish and mix with a spoon. Place in a 350degree oven and bake for 20 minutes. Add the garlic to the potatoes and mix. Cook for 15 minutes more. Take out of oven, and let set for five minutes before serving. Serve with any of the fish, meat, or poultry dish in the book.

Stuffed Mushroom

Prep Time: 10 min
Cook Time: 20 min
Servings: 4

INGREDIENTS
- Nonstick cooking spray
- 12 large white stuffing mushrooms, cleaned and stems removed and reserved
- 2 garlic cloves, finely chopped
- 2 tablespoons chopped fresh parsley
- 4 tablespoons olive oil
- ¾ cup bread crumbs, plus extra for topping
- ½ cup grated Parmesan cheese, plus extra for topping
- Salt

DIRECTIONS
1. Preheat the oven to 400°F. Spray a baking sheet with cooking spray.
2. Finely chop the mushroom stems and place them in a mixing bowl. Add the garlic, parsley, oil, bread crumbs, Parmesan cheese, and salt. Mix all the ingredients well. The mixture should be moist, so add another drizzle of oil if needed.
3. Salt the inside of the mushroom caps and stuff the caps with the stuffing. Place the mushroom caps on the baking sheet and sprinkle the tops with a pinch of bread crumbs and Parmesan cheese. Bake for 20 minutes.

Italian Stewed Tomatoes

Prep Time: 30 min
Cook Time: 10 min
Servings: 9

INGREDIENTS
- 24 large tomatoes - peeled, seeded and chopped
- 1 cup chopped celery
- ½ cup chopped onion
- ¼ cup chopped green bell pepper
- 2 teaspoons dried basil
- 1 tablespoon white sugar

DIRECTIONS
1. In a large saucepan over medium heat, combine tomatoes, celery, onion, bell pepper, basil and sugar. Cover and Cook for 10 minutes, stirring occasionally to prevent sticking.

NUTRITION: Calories: 100 cal | Fat: 1 g | Sodium: 399.7 g | Carbs: 22.2 g | Sodium: 34.4 mg

Tomato Onion Quiche

Prep Time: 20 min
Cook Time: 1 hour and 15 min
Servings: 3

INGREDIENTS

- 1 sheet refrigerated pie pastry
- 1 cup shredded part-skim mozzarella cheese
- 1/2 cup sliced sweet onion
- 2 small plum tomatoes, seeded and thinly sliced
- 3 medium fresh mushrooms, thinly sliced
- 1/4 cup shredded Parmesan cheese
- 3 large eggs
- 1/2 cup half-and-half cream
- 1/2 tsp. ground mustard
- 1/2 tsp. dried basil
- 1/2 tsp. dried oregano
- 1/2 tsp. dried thyme

DIRECTIONS

1. Cut pastry sheet in half. Rewrap; refrigerate one half for using later. Roll out the remaining half into an 8-inch circle on a lightly floured surface. Move to a 7-inch pie plate; flute edges.
2. Layer tomatoes, onion and half of the mozzarella cheese in pastry. Sprinkle with mushrooms on top; layer with tomatoes, onion and the remaining mozzarella cheese. Dust with Parmesan cheese. In a small bowl, mix herbs, mustard, cream and eggs; spread over top.
3. Bake at 350° till a knife comes out clean after being inserted in the center, or for 45-55 minutes. Allow to stand for 10 minutes and start cutting.

Nutrition: Calories: 436 Calories | Total Carbohydrate: 26 g | Cholesterol: 265 mg | Total Fat: 26 g | Fiber: 2 g | Protein: 22 g | Sodium: 516 mg

---

Crispy Cauliflower

Prep Time: 20 min
Cook Time: 30 min
Servings: 4

INGREDIENTS

- 1 cauliflower
- 1¼ cups fresh bread crumbs
- ½ cup freshly grated Parmesan or Grana Padano cheese
- 2 large eggs, slightly beaten
- Nonstick cooking spray
- A teaspoon of salt to taste

DIRECTIONS

1. Preheat the oven to 375°F. Spray a baking sheet with cooking spray.
2. Trim the cauliflower in a way that only florets will be remain. In a medium saucepan, cover the cauliflower and salt with water. Bring to a full boil and cook the florets for 4 to 5 minutes.
3. While boiling the cauliflower, mix the bread crumbs and cheese in a medium bowl. Set aside.
4. Drain the cauliflower and rinse cold.
5. Dredge one floret at a time in the beaten egg. Coat the dredge floret in the bread crumb-cheese mixture. Place on the baking sheet.
6. Bake the florets for 25 minutes, turning midway for even cooking

Vegetables

Fried Peppers with Potatoes

Prep Time 15 min | **Cook Time** 20 min | **Servings** 4

- 1/3 cup olive oil
- 3 or 4 large bell peppers of mixed colors, cut into strips
- 3 medium potatoes, peeled and cut into ¼-inch strips
- 1 medium onion, thinly sliced
- 1 teaspoon salt
- 1 teaspoon dried oregano
- 1 tablespoon chopped fresh parsley

1. In a large skillet or sauté pan over medium-high heat, heat the oil. Add the peppers, potatoes, onion, salt, oregano, and parsley, stirring to combine.
2. Reduce the heat to medium and mix all the ingredients well, paying close attention that the potatoes do not stick to the pan (see tip). Adjust the heat accordingly.
3. Continue frying the peppers and potatoes, stirring frequently, until fully cooked, about 20 minutes. Add additional oil if necessary. Serve hot.

Asparagus With Fresh Basil Sauce

Prep Time 10 min | **Cook Time** 15 min | **Servings** 12

- 3/4 cup reduced-fat mayonnaise
- 2 tbsps. prepared pesto
- 1 tbsp. grated Parmesan cheese
- 1 tbsp. minced fresh basil
- 1 tsp. lemon juice
- 1 garlic clove, minced
- 1-1/2 lbs. fresh asparagus, trimmed

1. Combine the first 6 ingredients in a small bowl until incorporated. Chill until ready to serve.
2. Boil 12 cups water in a Dutch oven; cook asparagus, in batches, for 2-3mins without cover until tender-crisp. Take the asparagus out then put in ice water right away; drain. Pat the asparagus dry then serve with sauce.

NUTRITION: Calories: 72 Calories | Total Carbohydrate: 3 g | Cholesterol: 6 mg | Total Fat: 6 g | Fiber: 1 g | Protein: 1 g | Sodium: 149 mg

Italian Style Green Beans

Prep Time 15 min | **Cook Time** 10 min | **Servings** 8

- 1-1/2 pounds fresh green beans, trimmed
- 2 plum tomatoes, chopped
- 1 small red onion, thinly sliced
- 1 can (3.8 ounces) sliced ripe olives, drained
- 1/2 cup prepared Italian salad dressing
- Dash each salt and pepper

1. In a Dutch oven, add beans and water to cover, then bring water to a boil. Cook, covered, until tender yet still crispy for about 4 to 6 minutes then drain. Put in leftover ingredients and heat through.

NUTRITION: Calories: 103 Cal | Sodium: 423mg | Fiber: 3g | Total Carbohydrate: 9g | Protein: 2g protein | Total Fat: 7g fat |

Stewed Eggplant and Tomatoes

Prep Time: 25 min | **Cook Time:** 1 hour | **Servings:** 6

INGREDIENTS

- 2 to 3 tablespoons extra-virgin olive oil
- 1 large onion, chopped
- 1 eggplant, cut into 1/2-inch cubes
- 2 (28 oz. each) cans San Marzano tomatoes
- 1/8 teaspoon oregano
- 2 tablespoons parsley
- 1/4 cup fresh basil, chopped
- 1/2 cup Italian cheese, grated

DIRECTIONS

1. Coat a large skillet with olive oil; sauté onion and eggplant until slightly soft. Crush tomatoes by hand. Add tomatoes with juice, oregano, parsley, basil and cheese to skillet and simmer for about 1 hour. Add more cheese, if desired.

Eggplant Bruschetta

Prep Time: 10 min | **Cook Time:** 5 min | **Servings:** 8

INGREDIENTS

- 1 medium eggplant, peeled and cut into 1/4-inch slices
- 1/2 teaspoon salt
- 3 medium tomatoes, seeded and chopped
- 2 tablespoons minced fresh basil
- 1 cup shredded part-skim mozzarella cheese
- 2 tablespoons shredded Parmesan cheese

DIRECTIONS

1. In a colander over a plate, put eggplant slices; scatter salt and toss softly. Allow to sit for half hour. Wash and drain thoroughly. With cooking spray, coat each side of every slice. Put on broiler pan. Atop eggplant with cheeses, basil and tomatoes. Broil 6 inches from the heat for 5 to 7 minutes till cheese is melted and eggplant is soft.

NUTRITION. Calories: 68 Cal | Total Carbohydrate: 7g | Cholesterol: 9mg | Protein: 5g | Fat: 3g | Sodium: 242mg

Italian Peas

Prep Time: 10 min | **Cook Time:** 15 min | **Servings:** 6

INGREDIENTS

- 2 tablespoons olive oil
- 1 onion, chopped
- 2 cloves garlic, minced
- 16 ounces frozen green peas
- 1 tablespoon chicken stock
- Salt and ground black pepper to taste

DIRECTIONS

1. In a large skillet, heat the olive oil over medium heat. Cook, stirring frequently, until the onion is softened, about 5 minutes. Cook for another minute after adding the garlic. Stir in the frozen peas and stock. Salt & pepper to taste.
2. Cover the skillet and cook for another 6 minutes, or until the peas are soft.

NUTRITION: Calories 106Cal | Protein 4.2g | Carbohydrates 12.3g | Fat 4.8g | Cholesterol 0.1mg | Sodium 120.5mg

Vegetables

Italian Kale

Prep Time: 15 min | **Cook Time:** 20 min | **Servings:** 4

INGREDIENTS

- 1 bunch chopped fresh kale leaves
- 1/2 tsp. minced garlic
- 1 tbsp. olive oil
- 2 tablespoons balsamic vinegar
- 1 dash Salt and ground black pepper to taste

DIRECTIONS

1. Cook the kale in a large, covered saucepan until the leaves wilt over medium-high heat. Cover and toss in the garlic, olive oil, and vinegar once the kale has been reduced by half. Cook for another 2 minutes while stirring. Season to taste with salt and pepper.

NUTRITION: Calories 92.4 Cal | Protein 3.8g | Carbohydrates 12.6g | Fat 4.2g | Sodium 147.1mg

Eggplant Cutlets

Prep Time: 15 min | **Cook Time:** 10 min | **Servings:** 6

INGREDIENTS

- 2 large eggplants, cut into ¼-inch slices
- Salt
- 1 cup fresh bread crumbs
- ½ cup freshly grated Parmesan cheese
- 1 cup all-purpose flour
- 2 eggs, beaten
- Vegetable oil, for frying

DIRECTIONS

1. Salt both sides of the eggplant slices and allow to rest on paper towels for 5 minutes.
2. In a shallow dish, combine the bread crumbs and Parmesan cheese and blend well. Pour the flour into a separate dish.
3. Lightly dredge each eggplant slice in the flour, shaking off the excess. Dip each slice in the beaten eggs, then dredge in the bread crumb and cheese mixture. Set aside on a baking sheet.
4. In a large frying pan over medium-high heat, heat about 1 inch of oil until shimmering. Working in batches, add a few slices of eggplant. Cook until lightly browned, about 2 minutes per side. If browning too quickly, lower the heat. Transfer the browned cutlets to paper towels and continue with the rest of the slices.
5. Plate and serve hot.

Gnocchi

Prep Time: 2-3 hours | **Cook Time:** 30 min | **Servings:** 4

INGREDIENTS

- 7 small potatoes, peeled, cooked
- 1 egg
- 2 to 2 1/2 cups flour
- 4 quarts unsalted water
- Pasta sauce

DIRECTIONS

1. Peel and boil potatoes; drain and mash. Cool slightly. Add egg and flour to potatoes to form a soft dough. With hands, make a rope about 1/2-inch in diameter. Cut into 1/2-inch to 3/4-inch pieces. Place on a lightly floured surface to dry for 2 to 3 hours.
2. In a large pot, bring water to a boil. Cook gnocchi in boiling water to which a bit of olive oil has been added. Cook on medium-high until gnocchi has risen to the surface. Remove with a slotted spoon, drain and serve with your favorite pasta sauce.

Fish and Seafood

Venice Fish Fillets

Prep Time: 5 min
Cook Time: 20 min
Servings: 4

INGREDIENTS

- 1 medium green or yellow bell pepper, julienned
- 1 small onion, julienned
- 1 1/2 lb. of fresh or frozen cod fillets, thawed
- 1/2 cup of fat-free Italian salad dressing
- 1/2 tsp. of Italian seasoning
- 2 (14.5-oz) cans of diced tomatoes

DIRECTIONS

1. In a pan, cook the onions, green peppers, salad dressing, and Italian seasoning until the vegetables are tender. Stir the tomatoes in and add the fillets.
2. Bring to a boil. Reduce the heat; cover and simmer for 11-13 minutes, or until the fish flakes easily with a fork. Serve.

Fettuccini and Salmon

Prep Time: 15 min
Cook Time: 15 min
Servings: 4

INGREDIENTS

- 1 lb. fettuccini, cooked, drained
- 4 cups whipping cream
- 1/2 cup butter
- 8 to 12 ounces smoked salmon, julienned
- 1/4 cup fresh chives, minced
- Freshly ground pepper, to taste
- Garnish: Fresh parsley or tarragon

DIRECTIONS

1. Cook fettuccini according to package directions; drain and set aside.
2. In a medium saucepan, combine whipping cream and butter; cook over medium high heat until thick, glossy and reduced by half. Add salmon, chives and pepper. Cook, stirring gently for 1 minute. Pour sauce over hot, cooked fettuccini. Garnish with parsley or tarragon.

Peppered Mussels

Prep Time: 20 min
Cook Time: 5 min
Servings: 4

INGREDIENTS

- 2 1/4 pounds. (1 kg) mussels, scrubbed and debearded.
- 1 clove garlic.
- 4 tbsp. (60 ml) added virgin olive oil.
- 8 slices crusty bread, toasted (optional).
- fresh parsley, cut, to taste pepper.

DIRECTIONS

1. Heat oil in a frying pan. include entire clove of garlic as well as cook up until great smelling, however do not brownish.
2. Include mussels, cover, and also cook until they open up.
3. Throw out any type of mussels that have not opened. spray mussels kindly with newly ground pepper as well as parsley. mix well. Transfer to serving bowls. offer with toasted bread, if using.

Herb-Grilled Salmon

Prep Time 15 min **Cook Time** 15 min **Servings** 4

INGREDIENTS

- 4 salmon steaks, about ¾-inch thick
- ¼ cup of olive oil
- ¼ cup fresh basil leaves
- ¼ cup fresh mint leaves
- 3 tbsp. lemon juice
- 1 clove garlic, minced
- Sea salt and freshly ground pepper

DIRECTIONS

1. Combine olive oil, basil, mint, lemon juice. And garlic in the small mixing bowl. Beat until well mixed.
2. Salt and pepper salmon steaks. Place them, single layer, in a dish. Pour marinade over. Cover and refrigerate 1 hour, turning after 30 minutes.
3. Preheat grill.
4. Remove salmon from marinade, reserving marinade. Place on the hot grill, and cook for about 6–7 minutes. Apply reserved marinade, and turn fish. Cook for another 6–7 minutes until salmon flakes easily.
5. Serve with pasta and vegetables. Decorate with basil leaves.

Lobster Tail with Tomato Confit and Basil Oil

Prep Time 15 min **Cook Time** 20 min **Servings** 4

INGREDIENTS

- 24 little lobster tails.
- 1 oz. (30 g) fresh basil, or about 1 1/4 cups whole fallen leaves.
- 3.5 oz. (100 g) mixed eco-friendlies, For serving 3 tbsp. (40 ml) extra-virgin olive oil.

prep work: 1 hr.
Half an hour.
Cooking: 6 minutes

For tomato confit

- 2 1/2 lbs. (1.2 kg) ripe tomatoes, or about 6 1/2 huge 1 clove garlic, very finely sliced.
- 1/2 oz. (10 g) fresh thyme, or regarding 1/4 cup 2 tsp. (10 ml) extra-virgin olive oil.
- sugar.
- Salt and pepper.

DIRECTIONS

1. Shell lobster tails, making use of scissors to lower back. period with salt, pepper and several of oil and let them season.
2. Warmth stove to 175 ° F (80 ° C) and also line a baking sheet with parchment.
3. Have ready a bowl of ice water. Bring a pan of water to a boil. peel tomatoes, drop them in boiling water, and also pale them For 30 seconds. Transfer them quickly to ice water. Cut them into quarters, get rid of seeds, as well as lay tomatoes on baking sheet. season on both sides with thyme, garlic, and also a pinch each of salt, pepper and sugar. Bake For 1 hr.
4. Line one more frying pan with parchment and established four specific square cooking mold and mildews on it. Load them with rotating layers of tomatoes as well as lobster tails, finishing with a layer of tomatoes. raise oven temperature level to 300 ° F (150 ° C), transfer to stove, and also bake For 6 minutes
5. Have all set a dish of ice water. Bring a tiny pan of water to a boil and also pale basil leaves, 2 minutes stress as well as put them straight in ice water. return basil leaves to frying pan as well as utilize an immersion blender or food processor to mix them with continuing to be oil.
6. eliminate molds from stove and also offer lobster tails as well as tomatoes with basil oil, in addition to mixed environment-friendlies.

Filet of Sole Francese

Prep Time: 20 min
Cook Time: 30 min
Servings: 30

INGREDIENTS

- 3 lbs. Lemon Sole Filet, cut into 6 equal pieces (about 3 ½ to 4 ounces each per serving)
- Salt & Black Pepper
- 2-3 Large Eggs seasoned with Salt & Pepper and beaten
- 1 cup Flour
- ½ stick Butter
- 2 Lemons, cut 6 Nice Slices (for Garnish) off one Lemon, leaving ½ piece of
- lemon remaining
- 2 Tablespoons of fine Chopped fresh Italian Parsley, do not use Dry Parsley
- ¼ cup Dry White Wine
- ½ cup vegetable oil, for cooking fish

DIRECTIONS

1. Season the Sole Filets with Salt & Pepper. Place four in a bowl and dredge the fish in flour. Then shake off excess flour. You will have the oil heating in a in a large frying pan over medium heat.
2. Put floured sole-filets into beaten eggs. By this time the oil in the pan should be hot enough to cook the fish.
3. With tongs pick the fish out of the eggs and let excess egg drip off of fish back into the bowl the beaten eggs are in. Immediately put the fish into the hot oil 1 piece at a time. Depending on the size of your pan you may have to cook the fish in two batches. Cook the fish about 2 minutes per side. Remove from pan and set onto a warm serving platter.
4. Remove all the oil from the pan. Add wine and turn heat to high. Cook until the wine has reduced by half its volume. Squeeze the juice of 1 ½ lemons into the pan and cook at low heat for 20 seconds. Turn heat off. Put butter in pan with heat off and swirl pan in a circular motion to incorporate butter with pan juices.
5. Place one piece of Sole on each person's plate with whatever vegetables you decide you want to serve the Sole with. Put the sauce from pan over the Sole in 6 equal portions. Sprinkle some parsley over each piece of fish and garnish each filet with one lemon slice. Serve and Enjoy.

Italian Christmas Eel

Prep Time: 15 min
Cook Time: 50 min
Servings: 4

INGREDIENTS

- 1 ½ pounds EEL
- have fishmonger skin and gut the eel
- 1 cup Tomato Sauce
- 2 large Potatoes, peeled and cut in ¼" slices
- ¼ cup Raisins, soaked in hot water for 20 minutes to soften,
- then drain dry.
- 12 Cerignola Olives, seed and coarsely chopped
- ¼ cup Capers, rinsed Capers from Pantelleria if possible)
- 1/2 cup Olive Oil
- 3 tablespoons top quality Italian Red Wine Vinegar
- 1/2 teaspoon Red Pepper flakes
- 1 clove Garlic, peeled and minced
- Salt & Black Pepper
- 4 tablespoons fresh chopped Parsley

DIRECTIONS

1. Put potatoes in a pot with water. Bring water to the boil. Once the water has come to the boil, lower to simmer and cook the potatoes for exactly 1 minute. Immediately remove potatoes from heat, drain, and set aside.
2. Heat tomato sauce in a small.
3. Cut eel into 3 inch pieces.
4. Line a large glass or ceramic casserole with a coating of olive oil. Neatly arrange all potatoes on bottom of casserole. Season the potatoes with Salt and ground Black Pepper.
5. Arrange all of the eel neatly on top of the potatoes. Dollop a tablespoon of tomato sauce over each piece of Eel. Lightly sprinkle olive oil over eel. Roast the EEL in a 375 degree oven for about 35 minutes until the eel is cooked through.
6. While the eel is cooking mix the chopped Olives, Capers, Garlic, Vinegar, 8 tablespoons Olive Oil, Red Pepper, 2 tablespoons Parsley, Raisons, Salt & Pepper to taste. Mix in a small glass mixing bowl and set aside.
7. Remove eel from oven and let cool down about 10 minutes before serving. Plate up the eel by putting 2 slices of potatoes on each person's plate. Set 1 piece of eel over the potatoes for each person. Spoon Olive Capers Sauce over top of each Eel and sprinkle on a pinch of remaining Parsley over each person's eel. Eat and enjoy and Buon Natale.

Fish and Seafood

Combined Fried Fish

Prep Time 5 min | **Cook Time** 30 min | **Servings** 4

- sea bream or sea bass, 2 lbs., 3 oz. (1 kg).
- 10 1/2 oz. (300 g). potatoes.
- oz. (50 g) Pecorino cheese, grated, or about 1/2 mug.
- 1 clove garlic, minced 1 tablespoon. sliced fresh.
- parsley.
- 3 tbsp. (40 ml) additional virgin olive oil.
- Salt and pepper.

1. Tidy squid by removing skin from body and also cutting arms from body. Flip back arms as well as squeeze out and also throw out beak located in center of tentacles. eliminate eyes, entrails, as well as transparent internal cartilage material. Cut body of squid right into rings (if squid is tiny, it can even be left whole).
2. prepare and fillet red mullet, intestine anchovies and sardines, and clean shellfishes, getting rid of heads.
3. heat oil in a big skillet up until hot. Dip various sorts of fish in semolina flour and also fry them independently, seeing to it that oil does not get too hot. eliminate fish from oil with a skimmer as well as dry theoretically towels. season with a pinch of Salt and also serve.

Cioppino

Prep Time 10 min | **Cook Time** 45 min | **Servings** 13

- 3/4 cup butter
- 1/2 teaspoon dried oregano
- 2 onions, chopped
- 1 cup water
- 2 cloves garlic, minced
- 1 1/2 cups white wine
- 1 bunch fresh parsley, chopped
- 1 1/2 pounds large shrimp - peeled and deveined
- 2 (14.5 ounce) cans stewed tomatoes
- 1 1/2 pounds bay scallops
- 2 (14.5 ounce) cans chicken broth
- 18 small clams
- 2 bay leaves
- 18 mussels, cleaned and debearded
- 1 tablespoon dried basil
- 1 1/2 cups crabmeat
- 1/2 teaspoon dried thyme
- 1 1/2 pounds cod fillets, cubed

1. Over medium-low heat melt butter in a large stockpot, add onions, garlic and parsley. Cook slowly, stirring occasionally until onions are soft.
2. Add tomatoes to the pot (break them into chunks as you add them). Add chicken broth, bay leaves, basil, thyme, oregano, water and wine. Mix well. Cover and simmer 30 minutes.
3. Stir in the shrimp, scallops, clams, mussels and crabmeat. Stir in fish, if desired. Bring to boil. Lower heat, cover and simmer 5 to 7 minutes until clams open. Ladle soup into bowls and serve with warm, crusty bread.

Nutrition: Calories: 318 Cal | Carbohydrates: 9.3g | Fat: 12.9g | Protein: 34.9g | Cholesterol: 164mg

Deviled Shrimp

Prep Time 5 min | **Cook Time** 15 min | **Servings** 4

- 2 tablespoons olive oil
- ½ small onion, chopped
- 2 garlic cloves, minced
- 2 cups canned crushed tomatoes
- Red pepper flakes
- 3 tablespoons chopped fresh parsley
- ½ cup water
- 1 pound medium shrimp, shelled and deveined

1. In a medium sauté pan over low heat, combine the oil and onion and cook, stirring occasionally, until the onion is translucent, 3 to 4 minutes.
2. Add the garlic, stirring to make sure it does not burn. Stir in the tomatoes, red pepper flakes to taste, parsley, and water. Increase the heat to medium and cook the sauce, uncovered, for 10 minutes.
3. Add the shrimp and cook them, stirring occasionally, until they turn pink, 4 to 5 minutes. Serve with pasta or with crusty bread.

Creamy Presto Shrimp

Prep Time: 15 min
Cook Time: 15 min
Servings: 8

- 1 pound linguine pasta
- 1 cup grated Parmesan cheese
- 1/2 cup butter
- 1/3 cup pesto
- 2 cups heavy cream
- 1 pound large shrimp, peeled and deveined
- 1/2 teaspoon ground black pepper

1. Bring a big saucepan of water to a boil. Cook for 8 to 10 minutes, or until al dente, with the linguine pasta; drain.
2. Melt the butter over medium heat in a large skillet. Season with pepper before adding the cream. Cook, stirring regularly, for 6–8 minutes.
3. Stir in the Parmesan cheese until it's well combined with the cream sauce. Cook for 3–5 minutes until the pesto has thickened.
4. Cook for 5 minutes, frequently stirring, until the shrimp turn pink. Serve with linguine that has been heated through.

NUTRITION: Calories: 646 | Carbohydrates: 43g | Fat: 42.5g | Protein: 23.1g | Cholesterol: 210mg

Monkfish in Leek Sauce with Italian Olives

Prep Time: 40 min
Cook Time: 25 min
Servings: 4

- 3 1/3 pound. (1.5 kg) monkfish.
- 5 tbsp. (70 ml) extra-virgin olive oil 7 oz. (200 g) ripe tomatoes, halved 1 lb. 2 oz. (500 g) leeks.
- 2 cloves garlic, cut.
- 1 bunch fresh parsley, sliced 1 pound. 2 oz. (500 g) olives.
- 3 mugs (700 ml) water.
- 4 tsp. (20 ml) white vinegar smashed red pepper flakes.

1. Salt as well as fresh ground pepper eliminate head, skin and also tail from monkfish as well as clean it thoroughly utilizing a sharp blade, fillet fish as well as get rid of main bone to acquire 2 fillets. Trim leeks, remove as well as discard dark environment-friendly components, as well as slice white as well as light eco-friendly parts right into rounds. rinse well under running water.
2. Bring a Saucepan of well-salted water to a boil. Pale leeks in water and also vinegar For a couple of seconds, drain and also dry.
3. Bring another pot of well-salted water to a boil. Cut monkfish fillets into uniform pieces, pale For a few minutes, drain, as well as reserved warmth oil in a skillet over medium warmth. include leeks and garlic as well as chef till softened. add a pinch of chile flakes, tomatoes, and also parsley, and offer a boil. add monkfish and olives. lower warmth to reduced and cook For 15 minutes period with Salt and also newly ground pepper and offer.

Bluefish Alla Lucia

Prep Time: 15 min
Cook Time: 20 min
Servings: 4

INGREDIENTS

- 4 Bluefish Filets 7-8 ounces each
- 1/3 cup Olive Oil
- Sea Salt & Black Pepper to taste
- 1 cup Tomato Sauce
- 3 cloves Garlic, peeled and sliced
- 3 Anchovy Filets, minced, 4 tablespoons Capers
- ¼ cup small Black Olives, pits removed
- ¼ cup fresh chopped Parsley

DIRECTIONS

1. Place a thin film of olive oil in a medium sized glass or ceramic baking dish. Add the bluefish to the pan. Sprinkle with a little Sea Salt & Black Pepper, and drizzle with olive oil.
2. Bake the Bluefish in a 350 degree oven until they are cooked through to the center, about 16 minutes.
3. Make the sauce by putting the remaining olive oil in a small frying pan with the garlic and anchovies. Cook on medium heat for 3 minutes. Add tomato sauce to pan with the Olives, Capers, and add half the Parsley. Cook 5 minutes on medium heat.
4. Remove Bluefish from the oven and let rest for 5 minutes before serving. Plate the fish onto 4 plates with a quarter slice of Lemon each. Pour a little sauce over each fish, and sprinkle with Parsley. Serve with whatever vegetable you like and enjoy.

Fish and Seafood

Almond and Pistachio-crusted Brownish-yellow Jack Steak with Artichoke Salad

Prep Time: 40 min
Cook Time: 1 hour
Servings: 4

INGREDIENTS

- 1 pound. (500 g) amberjack steaks or mahi 1 1/2 oz. (40 g) capers, or concerning 4 1/2 tbsp.
- 1/2 oz. (100 g) blanched almonds
- 3 1/2 oz. (100 g) pistachios
- 1 pound. 5 oz. (600 g) artichokes.
- 1 bunch fresh mint, carefully cut 2 lemons.
- 1/3 cup plus 1 1/2 tablespoon. (100 ml) extra-virgin olive oil Salt and pepper.

DIRECTIONS

1. Warmth oven to 350 ° F (180 ° C). Juice lemons, and include fifty percent of juice to a dish of water. get rid of challenging outer leaves from artichokes. Cut them in half as well as eliminate and dispose of chokes. slice artichokes really thinly as well as place them in lemon water to prevent staining.
2. Squash pistachios and almonds as well as spread them in a shallow dish. Cut fish crosswise right into thick pieces as well as layer them in crushed nuts.
3. In a blender or food processor, mix capers with 3 1/2 tbsp. (50 ml) of extra-virgin olive oil and get.
4. In a heatproof frying pan, warm a quarter of staying oil over tool warmth. scorch fish over tool warmth, period with Salt and transfer to oven. Cook For 5-10 minutes, depending on size of slices.
5. Drain pipes artichokes as well as throw them with remaining lemon juice, staying oil, and mint, as well as season to taste with Salt and pepper.
6. Serve fish with artichoke salad and also caper oil.

Nutrition: Calories: 436 Calories | Total Carbohydrate: 26 g | Cholesterol: 265 mg | Total Fat: 26 g | Fiber: 2 g | Protein: 22 g | Sodium: 516 mg

---

Garlic-and-herb-braised Squid

Prep Time: 15 min
Cook Time: 25 min
Servings: 12

INGREDIENTS

- 1 1/2 lbs. cleaned squid
- 2 cups flat-leaf parsley sprigs, divided
- 5 garlic cloves
- 3 tbsps. olive oil
- 1/4 tsp. hot red-pepper flakes
- 3/4 cup Chardonnay
- 1 (28-oz.) can whole tomatoes in juice, coarsely chopped
- 1/4 cup water
- Accompaniment: crusty bread

DIRECTIONS

1. Rinse squid in cold water. Pat dry. Cut big tentacles to half, lengthwise. Cut bodies and flaps, if they're there, to 1/2-inch- wide rings, crosswise.
2. Chop parsley to get 2 tbsp. Put aside. Chop leftover garlic and parsley together. In a 4-quart heavy pot, heat oil over low heat until hot. Cook red pepper flakes and garlic-parsley mixture for about 2 minutes, mixing, until garlic starts to sizzle. Bring heat up to medium-high, add the squid, for about 1 minute, cook and stir occasionally until it is barely opaque. Put the wine, simmering briskly and occasionally stirring, uncovered, for about 10 minutes until it reduces slightly. With their juice add tomatoes, 1/2 tsp. pepper, 1 1/4 tsps. salt, and water. Simmer, occasionally stirring, covered, for 30-40 minutes until squid is very tender.
3. Season with extra pepper and salt. Stir in leftover parsley.

NUTRITION: Calories: 221 | Total Carbohydrate: 11 g | Cholesterol: 264 mg | Total Fat: 9 g | Protein: 19 g

Cod with Potatoes

Prep Time 15 min **Cook Time** 30 min **Servings** 4

- 3 tablespoons olive oil
- 2 or 3 garlic cloves, sliced
- 2 to 3 tablespoons chopped fresh parsley
- 1 teaspoon dried oregano
- 2 cups canned crushed tomatoes
- 3 medium potatoes, peeled and diced
- 2 cups water, divided
- Salt
- 1½ pounds cod loins

1. In a large sauté pan over medium heat, combine the oil, garlic, and parsley. Cook for about 1 minute, just long enough to heat up the oil.
2. Add the oregano and tomatoes and cook for 5 minutes.
3. Add the potatoes and 1 cup of water, and cook for an additional 5 minutes. Add salt to taste.
4. Add the cod loins to the pan with the remaining 1 cup of water. Simmer, uncovered, for 20 minutes, until the broth has thickened. Serve with crusty bread or pasta.

Swordfish in Red Sauce

Prep Time 5 min **Cook Time** 25 min **Servings** 4

- 3 tablespoons olive oil
- ½ medium onion, diced
- 2 tablespoons chopped fresh parsley
- 3 garlic cloves, halved
- 1 teaspoon salt
- 1½ pounds swordfish, cut into large chunks
- 1 (28-ounce) can crushed tomatoes
- 1 cup water

1. In a large sauté pan over low heat, heat the oil, onion, parsley, garlic, and salt, and simmer for a few minutes, making sure the garlic does not burn.
2. Add the swordfish and allow it to brown for several minutes on each side. Remove and discard the garlic pieces.
3. Add the tomatoes and water, and simmer, uncovered, for 20 minutes, stirring a few times during the cooking process.

White Bean Crostini

Prep Time 15 min **Cook Time** 25 min **Servings** 12

- 1/8 tsp. pepper
- 1/4 tsp. salt
- 2 garlic cloves
- 1/4 cup plus 2 tbsp. olive oil
- 2 tbsp. minced fresh thyme or 2 tsp. dried thyme
- 2 tbsp. chopped ripe olives
- 1 can (15-oz) white kidney
- 24 slices French bread baguette (1/2 inch thick)

1. Put together the pepper, salt, garlic, 1/4 cup oil, and beans in a food processor. Put cover and process till smooth. Next, put thyme and olives; process till blended.
2. On an ungreased baking sheet, put the bread. Brush with leftover oil. Let broil 3 to 4 inches from the heat source for 1 to 2 minutes till golden brown. Slightly cool down. Scatter 1 tbsp. Bean mixture on each slice. Jazz up with thyme and olives if wished.

Fish and Seafood

Mediterranean Style Salmon

Prep Time 10 min | **Cook Time** 25 min | **Servings** 4

INGREDIENTS

- 1 pound cherry tomatoes, halved
- ¼ cup olive oil, plus more for baking dish
- 2 garlic cloves, halved
- 1 teaspoon dried oregano
- ½ teaspoon salt
- 4 salmon fillets
- Salt
- Freshly ground black pepper
- ½ cup black olives, pitted
- 2 tablespoons capers, rinsed

DIRECTIONS

1. In a medium bowl, combine the tomatoes, oil, garlic, oregano, and salt, and mix well. Let stand for 20 minutes.
2. In the meantime, wash the salmon and remove any skin.
3. Preheat the oven to 375°F. Add a few tablespoons of oil to a baking dish. Spread the tomatoes in the dish and top with the salmon.
4. Season with salt and pepper. Add the olives and capers on top and bake for 20 to 25 minutes. During baking, scoop some of the tomatoes on top of the fish. Serve immediately.

Spicy Shrimp & Peppers With Pasta

Prep Time 20 min | **Cook Time** 45 min | **Servings** 4

INGREDIENTS

- 1 cup sliced baby portobello mushrooms
- 1 medium sweet yellow pepper, cut into 1/2-inch pieces
- 1 medium green pepper, cut into 1/2-inch pieces
- 1 shallot, minced
- 2 tbsps. olive oil
- 1 garlic clove, minced
- 1/2 tsp. crushed red pepper flakes
- 1 can (28 oz.) crushed tomatoes
- 1 tsp. Italian seasoning
- 1/2 tsp. salt
- 6 oz. uncooked whole wheat linguine
- 1 lb. uncooked medium shrimp, peeled and deveined
- 3 tbsps. minced fresh parsley or 1 tbsp. dried parsley flakes

DIRECTIONS

1. Coat a big nonstick skillet with cooking spray. Sauté the mushrooms, shallot and peppers in oil until softened. Stir in pepper flakes and garlic; let it cook for additional 1 minute.
2. Add in the Italian seasoning, tomatoes and salt; stir. Allow the mixture to boil. Lessen the heat; make it to a simmer without any cover for 12-15 minutes or until vegetables are softened.
3. Meanwhile, prepare the linguine and cook following the package directions. Drop the shrimp to sauce; let it cook and stir for roughly 5-7 minutes or until it turns pink.
4. Drain the linguine and toss it into the sauce. Heat well. Top it off with parsley.

Baked Clams Oreganata

Prep Time: 20 min | **Cook Time:** 15 min | **Servings:** 13

INGREDIENTS

- ¼ cup finely chopped fresh Italian parsley
- ½ cup dry white wine
- ½ cup finely chopped red bell pepper
- ½ teaspoon kosher salt
- 1 teaspoon dried oregano, preferably Sicilian on the branch
- 1½ cups fine dried bread crumbs
- 36 littleneck clams, shucked, juices reserved
- 6 tablespoons extra-virgin olive oil
- Lemon wedges, for serving (not necessary)

DIRECTIONS

1. Preheat your oven to 425 degrees. As you shuck the clams, set them aside and reserve and strain their juices. Coarsely cut the shucked clams, and put in a large container. Put in the bread crumbs, bell pepper, 2 tablespoons parsley, the oregano, and salt. Sprinkle with 2 tablespoons olive oil, and toss using a fork to combine.
2. Stuff the clamshells with the filling, and place on a rimmed baking sheet; pour any extra juice, along with the white wine, into the bottom of the pan. Sprinkle the clams with 3 tablespoons olive oil, and sprinkle the rest of the tablespoon oil and rest of the 2 tablespoons chopped parsley into the bottom of the pan. Bake until the clam stuffing is browned and crunchy, approximately fifteen minutes. To serve: set the clams on a plate with rest of the sauce and fresh lemon wedges for squeezing (if using).

Piccata Cod

Prep Time: 10 min | **Cook Time:** 15 min | **Servings:** 4

INGREDIENTS

- ½ teaspoon ground black pepper
- 1 teaspoon paprika
- ½ teaspoon rosemary
- 2 tablespoon olive oil
- ½ teaspoon minced garlic
- 1 lemon
- 2 tablespoon capers
- 1-pound cod
- 1 teaspoon salt
- 3 tablespoon fresh parsley, chopped
- 5 tablespoon chicken stock
- 1/3 cup almond flour

DIRECTIONS

1. Squeeze the juice from the lemon.
2. Rub the cod with the salt and ground black pepper.
3. Combine the paprika with the rosemary, and almond flour. Stir the mixture.
4. Coat the cod fillet in the almond flour mixture.
5. Pour the olive oil into the pan and roast the cod for 3 minutes from the both sides.
6. When the fish is cooked – transfer it to the serving plate.
7. Then add the lemon juice to the remaining olive oil.
8. Sprinkle it with the capers, fresh parsley, minced garlic, and chicken stock.
9. Sauté the mixture until you get a thick sauce.
10. Then sprinkle the cooked cod with the sauce and serve it immediately.

NUTRITION: Calories 154 Cal | Fat 7.7g | Fiber 1g | Carbohydrates 2.88g | Protein 18g

Fish and Seafood

Meat
(Poultry, Beef, Pork and Lamb)

Lemon Chicken

Prep Time: 10 min
Cook Time: 45 min
Servings: 13

INGREDIENTS
- 1 cup fresh lemon juice
- 1 cup extra-virgin olive oil
- 1 tbsp. red wine vinegar
- 1 clove garlic, peeled and minced
- 1/2 tsp. dried oregano
- Salt and freshly ground black pepper
- 1/4 cup chopped fresh parsley
- 1 Broiler Chicken, cut into 10 pieces; 2 wings, 2 legs,
- 2 thighs, and cut the 2 breast in half making 4 pieces

DIRECTIONS
1. Season the chicken pieces with slat & black pepper.
2. Place all ingredients except the chicken, a quarter of the olive oil, and the parsley in a large glass or ceramic bowl. Set aside
3. Turn oven on to 450 degrees.
4. Put a large frying pan that will be large enough to hole all the chicken on stove top. Turn heat on high. Add ¼ of the olive oil to frying pan. Heat 2 minutes, then add the chicken.
5. Brown chicken in frying pan for 12 minutes, turning the chicken pieces every 4 minutes or so until nicely browned. Place chicken in oven and cook for 15 minutes.
6. Add the lemon mixture to pan with chicken. Return to oven and cook for 12 minutes.
7. Remove chicken from oven and peek into the inside of the chicken with a knife to make sure the chicken is cooked through and there is no blood. If there is blood, put chicken back in oven and let cook more until there is no more sign of blood on inside of chicken.
8. Place chicken on a place and keep warm in the oven turned down to 250 degree. Set frying pan with lemon juice mixture from chicken on top of the stove and cook over high heat for minutes. Remove from flame. Let cool down to warm for 5 minutes, then pour a little of the sauce over chicken and set the rest of the lemon sauce on the side. Sprinkle the fresh chopped Parsley over the chicken, serve and enjoy.

Zucchini and Corn-stuffed Chicken

Prep Time: 20 min
Cook Time: 53 min
Servings: 2

INGREDIENTS
- 1 small zucchini, finely chopped
- 1/4 cup fresh or frozen corn, thawed
- 3 tbsp. Parmesan cheese, grated, divided
- 2 boneless skinless chicken breast halves (6-oz each)
- 1 tsp. olive oil
- 1/8 tsp. salt
- 1/8 tsp. pepper

DIRECTIONS
1. Mix 2 tbsp. Cheese, corn, and zucchini in a small bowl. Slice a pocket in each chicken breast; stuff with half cup zucchini mixture on each pocket. Use toothpicks to secure.
2. Move to a cooking-spray-coated 8-inch square baking dish. Drizzle with oil, then scatters salt, remaining cheese, and pepper. Scoop the rest of the zucchini mixture surrounding the chicken. Bake for 30-35mins in a 350 degrees F oven without a cover or until a thermometer registers 170 degrees F.

Sausage, Peppers, Onion, And Potato Bake

Prep Time 15 min **Cook Time** 40 min **Servings** 8

INGREDIENTS

- 2 teaspoons olive oil
- 3 large onions, cut into wedges
- 2 pounds Italian sausage, sliced to 2-inch cuts
- 1/2 cup white wine
- 1/4 cup olive oil
- 1/2 cup chicken stock
- 4 large potatoes, peeled and thickly sliced
- 1 teaspoon Italian seasoning
- 2 seeded and cut into wedges huge green bell peppers
- season with salt and pepper to taste
- 2 seeded and cut into wedges huge red bell peppers
- 3 onions, peeled and sliced into wedges

DIRECTIONS

1. Preheat the oven to 400 degrees Fahrenheit (200 degrees C).
2. In a large skillet, heat 2 tablespoons olive oil over medium heat and brown the sausage, stirring occasionally. In a large baking dish, place the cooked sausage.
3. Pour 1/4 cup olive oil into the skillet and cook the potatoes for about 10 minutes, turning occasionally. Place the potatoes in the baking dish with a little oil left over.
4. In a heated skillet, cook and toss the green and red peppers and onions until they begin to soften, about 5 minutes. Fill the baking dish with the vegetables. Over the veggies and sausage, pour the wine and chicken stock, and season with Italian seasoning, salt, and pepper. Combine the sausage, potatoes, and veggies in a small mixing bowl.

Braised Lamb Shanks

Prep Time 25 min **Cook Time** 1 hour and 20 min **Servings** 4

INGREDIENTS

- 4 Lamb Shanks
- 4 Carrots, peeled
- 2 stalks Celery, washed and cut to small dice
- 2 medium Onion, peeled and chopped fine
- 6 cloves garlic, Peeled and chopped fine
- ¼ teaspoon each: Salt &Black Pepper
- 1 cup dry Red Wine
- 2 – 28 ounce can crushed Italian Tomatoes
- 5 tablespoons Tomato Paste
- 2 Idaho Potatoes, peeled and cut to large chunks
- 2 sprigs fresh Rosemary, 2 Bay Leafs
- 2 cups water
- 1 – 10 ounce box frozen Peas

DIRECTIONS

1. Place olive oil in a 6-quart non-corrosive pot. Season lamb with salt & pepper. Place lamb in pot and brown over a medium-high flame until the lamb is browned on all sides, about 12 minutes.
2. Remove lamb from pot and set aside. Add celery to pot and cook on high heat until light brown, about 8 minutes.
3. Add onions and cook on medium heat for 5 minutes. Add garlic, lower heat and cook for 2 minutes.
4. Add the wine and cook on high heat until the wine is reduced by half of its original volume, about 7 minutes.
5. Add tomatoes, tomato paste, and water to the pot. Add the lamb back to the pot and bring the liquid to boil. As soon as the liquid starts boiling, lower the heat to low and let all simmer for 30 minutes.
6. Cut the peeled carrots into large chunks.
7. After the lamb has been cooking for 30 minutes add the Carrots to the pot. Cook 20 minutes more and add the potatoes, rosemary, and Bay Leafs to the pot.
8. Continue cooking on a low simmer until the lamb is tender, which should be about 25-35 minutes more for a total cooking time of about 1 hour and 20 minutes. Cook the peas in boiling salted water, then drain.
9. To serve, place one Lamb Shank along with some potatoes, carrots, and peas, and a bit of sauce, saving most of the sauce for pasta the next day.

Meat

Roast Sicilian Rabbit

Prep Time: 20 min
Cook Time: 1 hour and 15 min
Servings: 4

INGREDIENTS

- 1 young Rabbit, about 2 ¼ pounds
- ¼ cup Olive Oil
- 4 tablespoons Flour
- ¼ cup Dry White Wine
- 6 cloves Garlic, Peeled and left whole
- 3 sprigs Fresh Rosemary
- Sea Salt & Ground Black Pepper
- 2 large Baking Potatoes (Idaho)
- ¼ cup chopped fresh Parsley

DIRECTIONS

1. Remove four legs from the rabbit. After removing the legs, you will have the center loin and breast flaps left. Cut the flaps off and cut into 4 pieces. You know have the center loin left. Cut this into four pieces. Season all of the rabbit pieces with Salt & Black Pepper. Dredge the rabbit pieces in the flour, and shake off excess.
2. Place olive oil in a large frying pan and turn heat on. Cook the rabbit over medium heat until all the rabbit is nicely browned, about 10-12 minutes. Remove rabbit from pan and set aside in a bowl.
3. Leave the olive oil in the pan, add the potatoes and cook on high heat for 5 minutes. Add the onions and cook on low heat for 5 minutes. Add garlic cloves and cook on medium heat for 3 minutes.
4. Remove everything from pan, including the oil and pour over the rabbit in the bowl.
5. Pour wine into the pan. Turn heat on to high and deglaze the pan by scraping the bottom of the pan with a wooden spoon to dislodge the browned bits sticking to the bottom of the pan. Cook until the wine is reduced by half it original volume.
6. Add water to pan. Return the rabbit, potatoes, and onions to the pan with all the juices in the bowl. Add Rosemary. Turn heat on and bring to the boil. Cover the pan with a lid or some aluminum foil and bake covered in a 350 degree oven in the oven for 30 minutes.
7. Remove covering from pan and continue baking in the oven for 15 minutes more.
8. Place potatoes and a few pieces of rabbit on each of 3-4 plates, leaving the juices in pan. Put the pan on a burner on top of the stove and turn heat on high. Cook over high heat to reduce the sauce and make it a bit thicker if it needs it. Turn heat off.
9. Pour the sauce in equal portions over the rabbit. Sprinkle with chopped Parsley and serve.

Easy Beef Braciole

Prep Time: 10 min
Cook Time: 25 min
Servings: 4

INGREDIENTS

- ½ onion, chopped
- 2 tablespoons olive oil
- 1 (28-ounce) can crushed tomatoes
- 8 thin slices beef rump or bottom round
- Salt
- Freshly ground black pepper
- 8 thin slices deli-style salami or prosciutto
- 8 thin slices provolone cheese
- Parsley sprigs, stemmed
- ½ cup grated Parmesan cheese

DIRECTIONS

1. In a large sauté pan, sauté the onion in the oil for a few minutes. Add the tomatoes and simmer.
2. In the meantime, prepare the braciole by sprinkling the meat slices with salt and pepper.
3. Place a slice of salami or prosciutto and cheese on top of each slice of meat. Add a few sprigs of parsley, and sprinkle some Parmesan cheese on top.
4. Roll up the meat tightly and, using a long toothpick, secure the meat closed. Repeat with the remaining meat.
5. Add the 8 braciole to the simmering sauce and cook for 25 minutes. Be sure to remove the toothpick before plating and serving.

NUTRITION: Calories 290 Cal | Fats 21 g | Sodium 503 mg | Carbohydrates 2.6 g | Protein 22.9 g

Cube Steak Parmesan

Prep Time: 15 min
Cook Time: 45 min
Servings: 8

INGREDIENTS

- 3 tablespoons all-purpose flour
- 3 tablespoons vegetable oil
- 1/2 teaspoon salt
- 4 (4 ounce) beef cube steaks
- 1/4 teaspoon ground black pepper
- 1 1/4 cups canned tomato sauce
- 2 eggs
- 2 1/4 teaspoons white sugar
- 2 tablespoons water
- 1/2 teaspoon dried oregano, divided
- 1/3 cup crushed saltine crackers
- 1/4 teaspoon garlic powder
- 1/3 cup grated Parmesan cheese
- 4 slices mozzarella cheese
- 1/2 teaspoon dried basil
- 1/3 cup grated Parmesan cheese

DIRECTIONS

1. Preheat the oven to 350°F (180°C) (175 degrees C). Combine the flour, salt, and pepper in a small bowl. Whisk the eggs and water together with a fork in a separate bowl. Combine the cracker crumbs, 1/3 cup Parmesan cheese, and basil in a third bowl or shallow dish.
2. In a large skillet, heat the oil over medium heat. Coat the cube steaks with seasoned flour, then dip them in the egg mixture and then in the cracker crumb mixture. Place them in the skillet. Cook until browned lightly on both sides. In a greased casserole dish, arrange the steaks in a single layer.
3. In a preheated oven, bake for 25 minutes. Meanwhile, combine the tomato sauce, sugar, 1/4 teaspoon oregano, and garlic powder in a medium mixing bowl. When the 25 minutes are complete, pour the sauce over the steaks. Top each steak with mozzarella cheese and the remaining Parmesan cheese, as well as the oregano. Bake for 6 minutes more, or until the cheese has melted and the sauce is bubbling.

NUTRITION: Calories: 458 | Carbohydrates: 17.1g | Fat: 28.8g | Protein: 32.5g | Cholesterol: 153mg

Roasted Calabrian Chicken

Prep Time: 10 min
Cook Time: 30 min
Servings: 4

INGREDIENTS

- Nonstick cooking spray
- 8 boneless skinless chicken thighs
- 1 teaspoon salt
- 1 small onion, sliced
- 3 tablespoons olive oil
- 2 or 3 sprigs rosemary, leaves only
- 2 to 3 teaspoons dried oregano
- 2 or 3 medium potatoes, peeled and cubed
- 1 lemon, halved

DIRECTIONS

1. Preheat the oven to 375°F, and move the oven rack to the second-lowest position. Coat a baking sheet with cooking spray or a few additional tablespoons of oil.
2. In a large mixing bowl, combine the chicken thighs, salt, onion, oil, rosemary, oregano, and potatoes, and mix well using clean hands or two wooden spoons.
3. Squeeze the lemon over all the ingredients.
4. Spread the ingredients on the baking sheet, and bake until the chicken is fully cooked, about 30 minutes.

Meat

Chicken Fettuccini Alfredo

Prep Time 30 min **Cook Time** 30 min **Servings** 8

INGREDIENTS

- 6 skinless, boneless chicken
- 1 tablespoon salt
- breast halves - cut into cubes
- tablespoons butter, divided
- 3/4 teaspoon ground white
- pepper
- 4 cloves garlic, minced, divided
- 1 tablespoon Italian seasoning
- 1 pound fettuccini pasta
- 3 cups milk
- 3/4 cup grated Parmesan cheese
- 1 onion, diced
- 8 ounces shredded Colby Monterey Jack cheese
- 1 (8 ounce) package sliced mushrooms
- 1/3 cup all-purpose flour
- 3 roma (plum) tomatoes, diced
- 1/2 cup sour cream

DIRECTIONS

1. Combine the chicken, 2 tablespoons butter, 2 garlic cloves, and Italian seasoning in a large skillet over medium heat. Cook until the inside of the chicken is no longer pink. Remove the pan from the heat and set it aside.
2. Bring a large saucepan of lightly salted water to a boil. Cook for 8 to 10 minutes, or until pasta is al dente; drain.
3. Meanwhile, in a skillet, heat 4 tablespoons butter. Cook the onion, 2 garlic cloves, and mushrooms in a skillet until the onions are translucent. Cook for 2-3 minutes after adding the flour, salt, and pepper. Slowly pour in the milk and half-and-half, stirring constantly until the mixture is smooth and creamy. Stir in the Parmesan and Colby-Monterey Jack cheeses until they are completely melted. Combine the chicken, tomatoes, and sour cream in a mixing bowl. Serve over fettuccini that has been cooked.

Roast Chicken With Rosemary

Prep Time 10 min **Cook Time** 2 hours to 2 hours 30 min **Servings** 6

INGREDIENTS

- 1 (3 pound) whole chicken, rinsed
- 1 small onion, quartered
- salt and pepper to taste
- 1/4 cup chopped fresh rosemary

DIRECTIONS

1. Preheat oven to 350 degrees F (175 degrees C).
2. Season chicken with salt and pepper to taste. Stuff with the onion and rosemary. Place chicken in a 9x13 inch baking dish or roasting dish.
3. Roast in the preheated oven for 2 to 2 1/2 hours, or until chicken is cooked through and juices run clear. Cooking time will vary a bit depending on the size of the bird.

Nutrition: Calories: 291 | Carbohydrates: 1.3g | Fat: 17.2g | Protein: 30.8g | Cholesterol: 97mg

Italian Lamb

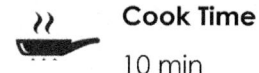

Prep Time: 20 min
Cook Time: 10 min
Servings: 4

INGREDIENTS

- 2 tbsp. of olive oil
- 1 lb. of lamb steak
- A handful of rosemary needles, chopped
- 8 oz. (250g) of British plum tomato
- 1 tbsp. of redcurrant jelly
- 2 tbsp. of capers, drained and rinsed
- 2 tbsp. of balsamic vinegar
- 3 oz. (100g) of feta cheese
- 3 oz. (100g) of British watercress
- Salt and black pepper
- Crusty bread to serve

DIRECTIONS

1. Toss the rosemary with 1 tablespoon of olive oil and marinate the lamb for 40 minutes. Wipe most of the rosemary out and season the steak with salt and black pepper. Sear the meat and tomatoes for about 3 minutes, or until golden, and set aside.
2. Whisk the vinegar, redcurrant jelly, and oil into a pan and warm until the dressing is made. Slice the lamb and spread the watercress and tomatoes on it, followed by cheese. Spoon over the sauce and serve with crusty bread.

Italian Stuffed Chicken Breast

Prep Time: 20 min
Cook Time: 50 min
Servings: 4

INGREDIENTS

- 1 ½ cups shredded Italian cheese blend
- 1 clove garlic, finely chopped
- 1 teaspoon dried basil
- 1 teaspoon dried oregano
- ½ cup grated Parmesan cheese
- ½ cup Italian-seasoned bread crumbs
- 4 pcs chicken breasts
- 1 beaten egg,
- 3/4 cup shredded Italian cheese blend (or as preferred)
- 1 cup homemade spaghetti sauce

DIRECTIONS

1. Preheat the oven to 350 degrees Fahrenheit (175 degrees C).
2. In a mixing bowl, combine 1 1/2 cup Italian cheese blend, garlic, basil, and oregano. In a separate bowl, combine the Parmesan cheese and bread crumbs.
3. Cut one side of each chicken breast horizontally down the centre to within a half-inch of the other. Open the two sides like a book and spread them out. To flatten the chicken, lightly pound it. Fill each chicken breast with the Italian cheese blend mixture and fold over the filling like a book. Wet the surface of chicken breast with beaten egg, then press the bread crumb mixture on top to coat each chicken breast. In a baking dish, arrange the chicken breasts.
4. Cook in a preheated oven for 45 minutes, or until the chicken is no longer pink in the middle and the juices run clear. An instant-read thermometer placed in the center should read at least 165 degrees F. (74 degrees C). Cover cooked chicken with 1/4 cup Italian cheese blend and spaghetti sauce. Bake for another 5 minutes, or until the cheese has melted and the sauce is boiling.

NUTRITION: Calories 470.1 Cal | Protein 43.5g | Carbohydrates 21.5g | Fat 22.7g | Sodium 1007.7mg

Meat

Lemon Chicken Piccata

Prep Time: 20 min
Cook Time: 25 min
Servings: 4

INGREDIENTS

- 3 large skinless, boneless chicken breast halves - cut into 1/2-inch medallions
- 1/2 lemon, thinly sliced
- salt and pepper to taste
- 1/4 cup fresh lemon juice
- 1/2 cup all-purpose flour
- 2 tablespoons capers, drained and rinsed
- 2 tablespoons vegetable oil, or as needed
- 3 tablespoons butter
- 1 clove garlic, minced
- 2 tablespoons minced Italian (flat-leaf) parsley
- 1 cup low sodium chicken broth

1. Preheat the oven to 200 degrees Fahrenheit (95 degrees C). To reheat a serving plate, place it in the oven.
2. Dredge the chicken breast pieces in flour after seasoning them with salt and pepper. Remove any excess flour by shaking it off. In a skillet, heat the vegetable oil and cook the chicken pieces until golden brown on both sides, about 3 minutes per side. Working in batches and not overcrowding the skillet as needed, add oil as needed. In the oven, place the chicken pieces on the warmed tray. Drain most of the oil from the skillet once all of the chicken has been cooked, leaving a thin coating on the pan's top.
3. In a skillet, cook and stir the minced garlic until fragrant, about 20 seconds. Add the chicken broth to the pot. Scrape any brown bits from the skillet's bottom and dissolve them. Bring the mixture to a boil after adding the lemon slices. Cook, stirring regularly, for 5 to 8 minutes, or until the sauce has reduced to about 2/3 cup. Add the lemon juice and capers and continue to cook for another 5 minutes, or until the sauce has reduced and thickened somewhat. Drop the butter into the skillet and swirl it into the sauce, turning the skillet to incorporate the butter. Remove from the pan and set aside the parsley.
4. Serve the chicken medallions on serving plates with sauce spooned over each portion

NUTRITION: Calories: 421 | Carbohydrates: 16.1g | Fat: 21.2g | Protein: 41.1g | Cholesterol: 128mg

Beef Braised in Barolo Wine

Prep Time: 30 min
Cook Time: 3 hour
Servings: 4

INGREDIENTS

- 3 1/3 lbs. (1.5 kg) beef chuck.
- 1 bottle Barolo red wine.
- 3 1/2 tbsp. (50 ml) extra-virgin olive oil.
- 2 cloves garlic, cut.
- 2 1/2 oz. (75 g) yellow onion, diced 2 oz. (60 g) carrot, diced.
- 2 stalks celery, diced.
- sprig fresh rosemary.
- 1 number fresh sage.
- 1 bay fallen leave.
- 1 clove.
- 1 cinnamon stick.
- 3-4 peppercorns salt.

DIRECTIONS

1. Link beef with kitchen area twine and placed it in a bowl with spices, herbs as well as vegetables.
2. add Barolo as well as marinade refrigerator For 12 hours get rid of meat and dry it. pressure out vegetables, reserving veggies and marinade. warm oil in a Dutch stove as well as sear meat. add reserved veggies and also remain to cook; after that include scheduled Sauce, season with salt, cover, and cook on low heat.
3. When meat is cooked, remove it from Dutch stove and allow awesome to make sure that it is much easier to cut. Meanwhile, placed Sauce through a veggie mill (or assimilate a food mill), stress it in a sieve, and also if required, reduce.
4. Cut beef right into thick pieces and immerse them in Sauce leave them there For some time to acquire flavor before serving.

Balsamic Vinegar Steak

Prep Time: 5 min **Cook Time:** 8 min **Servings:** 4

- ½ cup balsamic vinegar
- ¼ cup olive oil, plus 1 tablespoon, divided
- 1 teaspoon chopped fresh parsley
- 2 garlic cloves, minced
- 4 (5-ounce) boneless rib eye steaks, such as Delmonico
- Salt
- Freshly ground black pepper

1. In a small bowl, mix the balsamic vinegar, ¼ cup of oil, parsley, and garlic. Brush the steaks with the marinade, and season with salt and pepper.
2. In a large skillet over medium heat, heat the remaining 1 tablespoon of olive oil. When the oil is hot, add the steaks to the pan, reserving the remaining marinade. Cook the steaks to your desired doneness, 3 to 4 minutes per side for medium-rare.
3. Once cooked, remove the steaks from the pan and place them on a plate, covering them with aluminum foil.
4. Add the leftover marinade to the hot pan, cook for 2 to 3 minutes until the marinade is reduced by half. Uncover the steaks and pour the reduced glaze on top.

Chicken Milano

Prep Time: 10 min **Cook Time:** 15 min **Servings:** 4

- 2 cloves garlic, finely minced
- 4 half chicken breasts, boneless and skinless
- 1/2 teaspoon basil, crushed
- 1/8 teaspoon crushed red pepper flakes (optional)
- Salt and pepper, to taste
- 1 tablespoon olive oil
- 1 (14 1/2 oz.) can Italian style stewed tomatoes
- 1 (16 oz.) can Italian green beans, drained
- 1/4 cup whipping cream

1. Rub garlic over chicken. Sprinkle with basil and red pepper. Season to taste with salt and pepper, if desired. In skillet, brown chicken in oil. Stir in tomatoes. Cover and simmer 5 minutes. Uncover and cook over medium heat, 8 to 10 minutes, or until liquid is slightly thickened. Stir in green beans and whipping cream; heat through. Do not boil.

Parmesan Chicken Bake

Prep Time: 15 min **Cook Time:** 35 min **Servings:** 6

- 2 tablespoons olive oil
- 1/4 cup chopped fresh basil
- 2 cloves garlic, crushed and finely chopped
- 1 (8 ounce) package shredded mozzarella cheese, divided
- 1/4 teaspoon crushed red pepper flakes, or to taste
- 1/2 cup grated Parmesan cheese, divided
- 6 skinless, boneless chicken breast halves
- 1 (5 ounce) package garlic croutons
- 2 cups prepared marinara sauce

1. Preheat the oven to 350 degrees Fahrenheit (175 degrees C). Using olive oil, coat the bottom of a 9x13 inch casserole dish, then add garlic and spicy red pepper flakes.
2. Place the chicken breasts in the bottom of the dish and cover with marinara sauce. Over the marinara sauce, sprinkle basil and half of the mozzarella cheese, then half of the Parmesan cheese. Sprinkle the croutons on top, then finish with the remaining mozzarella and Parmesan cheese.
3. Bake for 35 minutes to an hour, depending on the shape and thickness of your chicken breasts, until the cheese and croutons are golden brown and the chicken is no longer pink inside. At least 160 degrees F should be read on an instant-read thermometer put into the thickest portion of a chicken breast (70 degrees C).

NUTRITION: Calories: 477 | Carbohydrates: 28g | Fat: 21.7g | Protein: 40.3g | Cholesterol: 100mg

Meat

Garlic Tomato Sauce and Meatballs

Prep Time
20 min

Cook Time
1 hour and 10 min

Servings
4

INGREDIENTS

Sauce:
- 3 to 4 tablespoons extra-virgin olive oil
- 1/2 cup onion, chopped
- 4 cloves garlic, minced
- 1 tablespoon fresh Italian parsley, chopped
- 1 (8 oz.) can tomato sauce + scant can of water
- 1 (6 oz.) can tomato paste + scant can of water
- 1 teaspoons dried oregano
- 1/4 teaspoon dried sweet basil
- 1 bay leaf
- 1/2 teaspoon dried Italian seasoning
- 1/2 teaspoon granulated sugar
- Salt and pepper, to taste

Meatballs:
- 1/2 lb. lean ground beef
- 1/4 lb. ground pork (optional)
- 2 cloves garlic, minced
- 1 egg, beaten
- 2 to 3 tablespoons water
- 1 cup plain dry breadcrumbs (add more as needed)
- 2 teaspoons Parmesan cheese, grated
- 1/4 teaspoon dried oregano
- 1/2 teaspoon fresh parsley, chopped
- 1/2 teaspoon salt
- 1/4 teaspoon peppe

DIRECTIONS

Sauce: Heat olive oil in a medium saucepan on high. Add onions and sauté 1 minute. Turn down heat to medium-high. Cook for 10 minutes or until beginning to brown. Add garlic, sauté about 5 minutes, or until both are golden brown (careful not to burn). Add fresh parsley and sauté just a few seconds. Add tomato sauce and paste. Fill cans with equal parts of water (scant) and add to sauce. Stir well until all lumps are dissolved. Add dried herbs by crushing between your hands. Add sugar, salt and pepper. Reduce heat to low and simmer 45 minutes to 1 hour. Add cooked meatballs.

Meatballs: Mix ground beef with ground pork until well blended. Add remaining ingredients and mix well. Shape into 1 1/2 to 2-inch balls. Heat skillet with about 1 to 2 tablespoons olive oil. Place meatballs in pan and cook over medium-high heat, turning when meat loosens from pan. When done, remove and drain on paper towels. Add to sauce, stirring carefully.

1. To serve with cooked pasta: Place drained pasta in a pot. Toss with 1/2 cup sauce, coating the pasta with a light coating of sauce. Serve on plates and drizzle with a little more sauce on top. Sprinkle and garnish with fresh chopped basil and grated Parmesan/Romano cheese. Place any leftover sauce in a sauceboat or server.

Buffalo Mozzarella and Semi-Candied Tomatoes

Prep Time 20 min **Cook Time** 1 hour and 10 min **Servings** 4

INGREDIENTS

- 1/4 lb. (120 g) puff pastry, or 1 sheet.
- 1 3/4 oz. (50 g) pancetta or thick bacon, diced 1/2 pound. (250 g) potatoes.
- 1/2 mug (125 ml) milk.
- 1 huge egg.
- 1 sprig fresh rosemary, leaves cut.
- Salt and pepper

DIRECTIONS

1. Warmth oven to 200 ° F (100 ° C). Cut tomatoes, and prepare them on a flat pan. Sprinkle with salt, a little sugar, garlic, as well as thyme. Drizzle with olive oil and cook for regarding an hour.
2. At same time, bring a tool pot of water to a boil. Dip basil in water and then plunge into ice water. Puree basil leaves in a blender or food processor with 3 1/2 tablespoon. (50 ml) olive oil. Slice mozzarella as well as period lightly with Salt and pepper.
3. Make heaps by layering mozzarella as well as semi-candied tomato slices. Drizzle with olive oil and garnish with basil Sauce.

Pork with Olives

Prep Time 10 min **Cook Time** 25 min **Servings** 4

INGREDIENTS

- 1 small pork tenderloin , cut into 1½-inch-thick rounds
- ½ cup flour
- Salt
- Freshly ground black pepper
- ¼ cup olive oil
- 3 sprigs rosemary , leaves only, stemmed
- 1 cup dry white wine
- ½ cup green olives , pitted and halved

DIRECTIONS

1. Gently coat the pork tenderloin pieces in the flour. Season with salt and pepper. Set aside. Step 2
2. In a large sauté pan over medium-high heat, heat the oil and rosemary for a few minutes. Step 3
3. Add the pork to the oil and brown on all sides. Add the white wine and olives.
4. Reduce the heat to low, and continue cooking the pork for an additional 15 to 20 minutes, uncovered. If the juices are drying up too quickly, reduce the heat and add a little bit of water. A little bit of juice should remain to top the meat with before serving.

Pan Chicken with Tomato

Prep Time 10 min **Cook Time** 15 min **Servings** 4

INGREDIENTS

- 3 tablespoons olive oil
- 2 garlic cloves, minced
- 1 pint cherry tomatoes, halved
- 1 teaspoon salt
- 1 pound chicken tenders, cut into 4 or 5 pieces
- 1 teaspoon dried oregano
- ¼ cup black or green olives, pitted

DIRECTIONS

1. In a large sauté pan over low heat, combine the oil and garlic, and cook for one minute. Add the tomatoes and salt, increase the heat to medium, and cook the tomatoes until they burst and cook down, about 5 minutes.
2. Add the chicken and oregano to the pan, mixing well. Add the olives.
3. Continue cooking until the chicken is no longer pink, about 10 additional minutes.

Meat

Italian Frittata ham

Prep Time: 10 min
Cook Time: 25 min
Servings: 14

INGREDIENTS

- 7 oz mushroom
- 1 cup milk
- 8 oz ham
- 1 teaspoon minced garlic
- 9 eggs
- 1 onion
- 1 cup cherry tomatoes
- 8 oz Parmesan
- 1 tablespoon basil
- 1 tablespoon dill
- ½ teaspoon paprika
- 2 tablespoon butter
- 1 tablespoon parsley
- ½ teaspoon salt

DIRECTIONS

1. Separate the egg yolk and egg white. Whisk the egg yolks until you get the lemon color of the mixture.
2. After this, whisk the egg whites till the strong peaks. Combine the egg yolks and egg whites together. Pour the milk and whisk it gently until homogenous.
3. Sprinkle the liquid with the paprika and salt. Then peel the onion and dice it.
4. Chop the ham. Toss the butter in the deep pan and melt it. When the butter is melted – put the diced onion inside. Cook it until the onion starts to be tender. Then add chopped ham and cook it for 3 minutes more.
5. Meanwhile, make the halves from the tomatoes. Add the tomato halves to the onion mixture.
6. Grate Parmesan cheese and slice the mushrooms. Add the sliced mushrooms to the pan and simmer the mixture for 4 minutes more. After this, add the minced garlic, dill, basil, paprika, and parsley in the egg mixture. Whisk it gently again.
7. Pour the egg liquid in the pan mixture and stir it. Sprinkle the dish with the grated cheese and close the lid. Reduce the heat to medium and cook the frittata for 3 minutes. After this, transfer the pan with the frittata in the preheated to 365 F oven. Cook the meal for 12 minutes more.
8. Then chill the prepared dish and serve it.

NUTRITION: Calories 236 | fat 9.8 | fiber 2 | carbs 21.05 | protein 17

Turkey Cutlets

Prep Time: 10 min
Cook Time: 25 min
Servings: 4

INGREDIENTS

- Salt and black pepper to the taste
- A pinch of paprika
- A pinch of cayenne pepper
- 2 eggs
- 4 turkey breast cutlets
- ¼ cup parsley, chopped
- 4 ounces feta cheese, crumbled
- ¼ cup red onion, chopped
- 1 and ½ cups couscous
- ½ cup vegetable oil
- 1 cup breadcrumbs
- 2 cups chicken stock
- 1 tablespoons sesame seeds
- ½ cup white flour
- 4 lemon wedges

DIRECTIONS

1. Heat up a pan with 2 tablespoon oil over medium high heat, add couscous, stir and cook for 7 minutes.
2. Add stock, bring to a boil, reduce heat to medium-low, simmer for 10 minutes, take off heat and keep warm.
3. In a bowl, mix breadcrumbs with sesame seeds, cayenne, paprika, salt and pepper.
4. Whisk eggs well in another bowl and put the flour in a third one.
5. Dredge turkey cutlets in flour, eggs and breadcrumbs and arrange them on the plate.
6. Heat up a pan with the rest of the oil over medium high heat, add cutlets, cook for 3 minutes flipping once and transfer them to paper towels in order to drain excess grease.
7. Mix couscous with parsley onion, salt, pepper and feta cheese and stir.
8. Divide turkey cutlets on plates, add couscous on the side and serve with lemon wedges.

NUTRITION: Calories 760 | Fat 20g | Fiber 4g | Carbohydrates 34g | Protein 40g

Lamb Stew With Mint And Apricots

Prep Time: 10 min
Cook Time: 1 hour
Servings: 4

INGREDIENTS

- 2 pounds lamb shoulder chops
- 1 tablespoon mustard, dry
- 3 tablespoons canola oil
- 1 tablespoon ras el hanout
- 1 carrot, chopped
- 3 cups orange juice
- ½ cup mint tea
- Salt and black pepper to the taste
- 1 yellow onion, chopped
- 1 celery rib, chopped
- 2-star anise
- 1 cup apricots, dried and cut in halves
- 1 cinnamon stick
- 1 tablespoon ginger, grated
- 28 ounces canned tomatoes, crushed
- 1 tablespoon garlic, minced
- ½ cup mint, chopped
- 15 ounces canned chickpeas, drained
- 6 tablespoons yogurt

DIRECTIONS

1. Put orange juice in a pot, bring to a boil over medium heat, take off heat, add tea leaves, cover and leave aside for 3 minutes, strain this and leave aside.
2. Season meat with salt and pepper, add mustard and ras el hanout and toss to coat.
3. Heat up a pot with 2 tablespoons oil over medium high heat, add lamb chops, brown for 3 minutes on each side and transfer to a plate.
4. Add the rest of the oil to the pot and heat it up.
5. Add ginger, onion, carrot, garlic and celery, stir and cook for 5 minutes.
6. Add orange juice, star anise, tomatoes, cinnamon stick, lamb, apricots, stir and cook for 1 hour and 30 minutes.
7. Transfer lamb chops to a cutting board, discard bones and chop.
8. Bring sauce from the pot to a boil, add chickpeas, stir and cook for 10 minutes.
9. Discard cinnamon and star anise, add mint, stir and divide into bowls.
10. Serve with yogurt on top.

Nutrition: Calories 560Cal | Fat 24g | Fiber 11g | Carbohydrates 35g | Protein 33g

---

Tunisian-Style Ribs

Prep Time: 10 min
Cook Time: 3 hours
Servings: 6

INGREDIENTS

- 1 cup carrots, chopped
- 1 cup figs, dried and chopped
- 1 tablespoon ginger, grated
- 3-star anise
- 1 tablespoon garlic, minced
- 2 cinnamon sticks
- 1 cup canned tomatoes, crushed
- 1 cup red wine
- 3 tablespoons vegetable oil
- 12 beef short ribs
- Salt and black pepper to the taste
- 1 cup onions, chopped
- 1 cup chicken stock
- ¼ cup soy sauce
- 2 tablespoons mint, chopped
- 2 tablespoons parsley, chopped

DIRECTIONS

1. Heat up a pot with 2 tablespoons oil over medium high heat, add short ribs, season with salt and pepper to the taste, cook for 4 minutes on each side and transfer to a plate.
2. Add the rest of the oil to your pot and heat up over medium high heat.
3. Add onions and carrots, salt and pepper, stir and cook for 8 minutes.
4. Add figs, ginger, garlic, cinnamon sticks, star anise, stir and cook for 1 minute.
5. Add ½ cup wine, stir and cook for 1 minute.
6. Return ribs to the pot, add tomatoes, soy sauce, the rest of the wine and stock, stir, bring to a simmer, cover and introduce in the oven at 325 degrees F.
7. Bake for 2 hours and 50 minutes, stirring gently every 40 minutes.
8. Add salt, pepper, parsley and mint, stir, divide into plates and serve.

NUTRITION: Calories 300 cal | Fat 23g | Fiber 4g | Carbohydrates 23g | Protein 35g

Meat

Great Meatloaf

Prep Time: 10 min
Cook Time: 1 hour and 20 min
Servings: 8

INGREDIENTS

- 4 ounces white bread, chopped
- 2 pounds lamb, ground
- 1 cup milk
- ¼ cup feta cheese, crumbled
- 2 eggs
- 1/3 cup kalamata olives, pitted and chopped
- 4 tablespoons oregano, chopped
- Salt and black pepper to the taste
- 2 tablespoons honey
- 1 tablespoon Worcestershire sauce
- 2 teaspoons lemon zest, grated
- 1 yellow onion, chopped
- 2 tablespoons olive oil
- 2 garlic cloves, minced
- ¾ cup red wine

DIRECTIONS

1. Heat up a pan with 2 tablespoons oil over medium heat, add garlic and onion, stir and cook for 8 minutes.
2. Add wine, stir, simmer for 5 minutes and transfer everything to a bowl.
3. Put bread pieces in a bowl, add milk, leave aside for 10 minutes, squeeze bread a bit, chop and add it to onions mix.
4. Add lamb, eggs, cheese, olives, lemon, zest, oregano, Worcestershire sauce, salt and pepper to onions mix and stir very well.
5. Transfer meatloaf mix to a baking dish, spread honey all over, introduce in the oven at 375 degrees F and bake for 50 minutes.
6. Take meatloaf out of the oven, leave aside for 5 minutes, slice and arrange on a platter.

Nutrition: Calories 350 Cal | Fat 23g | Fiber 1g | Carbohydrates 17g | Protein 24g

---

Italian Pork Tenderloin

Prep Time: 15 min
Cook Time: 35 min
Servings: 4

INGREDIENTS

- 1 ½ pounds pork tenderloin, cut into half inch strips
- 2 tbsp. olive oil
- ¼ cup chopped prosciutto
- 2 tbsp. fresh parsley
- 2 tbsp. fresh sage, chopped
- 2 tbsp. chopped sun-dried tomatoes
- 1/3 cup chopped onion
- 1/3 cup chicken broth
- ½ cup heavy cream
- ¼ tsp. salt
- ground black pepper to taste

DIRECTIONS

1. In a skillet, heat the oil over medium-high heat. 5 minutes, until the onion is soft, saute the prosciutto, sage, parsley, sun-dried tomatoes, and onion. In a skillet, combine the pork strips and cook for 10 minutes, stirring once.
2. Season with salt and pepper before adding the broth and heavy cream to the skillet.
3. Bring the water to a boil. Reduce heat to low and cook, stirring periodically, for 20 minutes, or until pork achieves a minimum temperature of 145°F (63°C) and sauce has thickened.

Nutrition: Calories 356 Cal | Protein 28g | Carbohydrates 3.1g | Fat 25g | Cholesterol 121.8mg | Sodium 390.3mg

Simple Braised Beef

Prep Time: 3 hours
Cook Time: 3 hours and 30 min
Servings: 6

INGREDIENTS

- For the ribs:
- 3 tablespoons olive oil
- 1 carrot, chopped
- 1 yellow onion, chopped
- 1 celery stalk, chopped
- 1 and ½ cups ruby port
- 2 bay leaves
- 6 beef short ribs
- 1 tablespoon thyme, chopped
- Salt and black pepper to the taste
- 2 and ½ cups red wine
- 2 tablespoons balsamic vinegar
- 6 cups beef stock
- 4 parsley springs
- For the salsa:
- 1 cup parsley, chopped
- 1 teaspoons marjoram, chopped
- ¼ cup mint, chopped
- 1 garlic clove, minced
- 1 tablespoons capers, drained
- 1 anchovy
- ¾ cup olive oil
- Salt and black pepper to the taste
- ½ cup feta cheese, crumbled

DIRECTIONS

1. In a bowl, mix thyme with salt and pepper, add short ribs, toss to coat and leave aside for 30 minutes.
2. Heat up a pot with the oil over high heat, add short ribs, sear for 3 minutes on each side and transfer them to a bowl.
3. Heat up the pan again over medium heat, add celery, onion, carrot and bay leaves, stir and cook for 8 minutes.
4. Add port, vinegar and wine, stir, bring to a boil and simmer for about 10 minutes.
5. Add stock, return short ribs, parsley, salt and pepper, cover and bake in the oven at 325 degrees F for 3 hours.
6. Take ribs out of the oven and leave aside for 30 minutes.
7. In your food processor, mix 1 cup parsley with marjoram, mint, 1 garlic clove, capers, anchovy, ¾ cup olive oil, feta cheese, salt and pepper and pulse well.
8. Divide short ribs into bowls, add some of the cooking liquid and tops with the salsa you've just made!

NUTRITION: Calories 450 Cal | Fat 45g | Fiber 2g | Carbohydrates 18g | Protein 43g

Spicy Sausage Linguine

Prep Time: 10 min
Cook Time: 10 min
Servings: 4

- 2 tbsps. olive oil
- 1 lb. fully cooked smoked sausages (such as hot links), cut diagonally into 1/4-inch-thick slices
- 1 large onion, chopped
- 6 large garlic cloves, minced
- 1 tsp. dried crushed red pepper
- 1 tsp. dried basil
- 1 tsp. dried oregano
- 1 tsp. rosemary
- 1 lb. linguine
- 1 1/2 cups canned low-salt chicken broth
- 1/4 cup freshly grated Parmesan cheese
- 2 tbsps. chopped fresh parsley

DIRECTIONS

1. On medium-high heat, heat oil in a big heavy pan. Sauté sausages in hot oil for 5mins until brown. Move sausages on paper towels using a slotted spoon to drain. In the same pan, sauté rosemary, chopped onion, oregano, minced garlic, basil, and dried crushed pepper for 5mins until the onion is golden. Put the sausage back in the pot; sprinkle pepper and salt. Take off heat.
2. In the meantime, in a big pot, cook pasta until tender yet still firm to chew in boiling water; drain. Add broth in the pot then boil. Toss the pasta back in the pot to coat.
3. Move broth and pasta to a big bowl. Scoop the sausage mixture on top of the pasta. Top with parsley and Parmesan cheese to serve.

NUTRITION: Calories: 878 | Carbohydrate: 94 g | Cholesterol: 84 mg | Fat: 39 g | Protein: 38 g | Sodium: 974 mg

Meat

Italian Barbeque Pork Chops

Prep Time: 10 min | **Cook Time:** 20 min | **Servings:** 4

INGREDIENTS
- ¾ cup balsamic vinegar
- ½ cup ketchup
- ¼ cup brown sugar
- 1 clove garlic, minced
- 1 tablespoon Worcestershire sauce
- 1 tablespoon Dijon mustard
- ½ teaspoon salt
- ½ teaspoon freshly ground black pepper
- 4 (6 ounce) pork loin chops
- 1 pinch salt and freshly ground black pepper to taste

DIRECTIONS
1. In a saucepan over medium-low heat, combine the balsamic vinegar, ketchup, brown sugar, garlic, Worcestershire sauce, Dijon mustard, 1/2 teaspoon salt, and 1/2 teaspoon black pepper; boil the sauce for 20 minutes. Allow to cool for 5 minutes after removing from the heat.
2. Preheat an outside grill to medium heat and brush the grate gently with oil. Season the pork chops on both sides with salt and black pepper. Brush the sauce from the saucepan over the chops.
3. Cook the pork chops on the prepared grill for about 5 minutes per side, or until the pork is no longer pink in the center. The temperature should read 145 degrees F on an instant-read thermometer put into the center (63 degrees C). Allow it rest for 3 minutes before serving with the remaining sauce on the side.

NUTRITION: Calories: 298 Calories | Carbohydrate: 30g | Fat: 6.6g | Protein: 22.4g | Sodium: 907.1mg

---

Beefy Italian Ramen Skillet

Prep Time: 10 min | **Cook Time:** 15 min | **Servings:** 5

INGREDIENTS
- 1 pound ground beef, or to taste
- 16 slices pepperoni, or to taste
- 1 (14.5 ounce) can diced tomatoes
- 1 cup water
- 2 (3 ounce) packages beef-flavored ramen noodles
- 1 green bell peppers, cut into strips
- 1 cup shredded mozzarella cheese

DIRECTIONS
1. In a large skillet, heat the oil over medium-high heat. 5 to 7 minutes, cook and toss beef and pepperoni slices in a heated skillet until beef is thoroughly browned. Toss the meat combination with tomatoes, water, and the contents of the ramen noodle spice container
2. .Break the ramen noodle blocks in half and add to the meat mixture with the green bell pepper; cook for 5 minutes or until the noodles soften.
3. Remove skillet from heat, sprinkle mozzarella cheese over the beef mixture, and cover; set aside for about 3 minutes, or until cheese has melted.

NUTRITION: Calories: 298 Calories | Carbohydrate: 7.4g | Fat: 18.4 6g | Protein: 23.4g | Sodium: 546.3mg

Quail Stuffed with Mushrooms and Sausage

Prep Time: 15 min **Cook Time:** 15 min **Servings:** 4

INGREDIENTS

- 1/3 cup freshly grated Grana Padano
- 1 bunch scallions, trimmed and chopped (approximately 1 cup)
- 1 celery stalk, finely chopped
- 1 pound mixed mushrooms, 4 ounces finely chopped, 12 ounces cut (button, cremini, shiitake, chanterelle, oyster)
- 1 small onion, finely chopped
- 1¼ teaspoons kosher salt
- 1½ cups dry white wine
- 1½ cups milk
- 2 links sweet Italian sausage (approximately seven ounces), removed from casings
- 2 tablespoons chopped fresh Italian parsley
- 2 tablespoons extra-virgin olive oil
- 4 cups crustless day-old country-bread cubes
- 6 tablespoons unsalted butter
- 8 semi-boneless quail (about 2 pounds)
- Freshly ground black pepper

DIRECTIONS

1. Preheat your oven to 400 degrees. Place the bread in a big bowl, and pour the milk over it. Let the bread soak while you assemble the stuffing for the quail. In a big frying pan on moderate heat, melt 2 tablespoons of the butter in the olive oil. When the butter is melted, put in the onion and celery. Cook until everything just starts to tenderize, approximately 4 minutes.
2. Raise the heat to moderate high, and put in the chopped mushrooms and sausage. Cook, breaking up the sausage using a wooden spoon, until the sausage and mushrooms are thoroughly browned, approximately three minutes. Put in the scallions, flavor with ½ teaspoon of the salt and some pepper, and cook until the scallions are wilted, approximately three minutes. Put in ½ cup of the white wine, and simmer quickly until the wine is reduced away, approximately two minutes. Scrape the mixture into a bowl to cool.
3. When the vegetables are cooled, squeeze the bread dry, leaving the milk in the bowl, and put in the bread to the vegetables, breaking it up using your fingers. Mix in the parsley and grated cheese, and mix thoroughly. Flavor the quail inside and out with ½ teaspoon salt and some pepper. Split the stuffing among the body cavities of the quail.
4. Heat a big roasting pan on moderate heat. Put in the rest of the 4 tablespoons butter. When the butter is melted, put in the cut mushrooms, and flavor with the rest of the ¼ teaspoon salt. Cook and stir until the mushrooms become tender, approximately six minutes. Put in the rest of the cup of white wine, and bring it to its boiling point. Set the quail, breast side up, on the mushrooms, and roast them until the skin is golden and the quail are thoroughly cooked, approximately half an hour. Adjust the pan sauce for seasoning. Serve the quail with the mushroom pan sauce ladled over the top.

Milan-Style Porkchops

Prep Time: 10 min **Cook Time:** 25 min **Servings:** 4

INGREDIENTS

- ½ cup all-purpose flour
- 2 cups bread crumbs
- 2 eggs, lightly beaten
- 1 cup clarified butter, divided
- 4 bone-in pork chops
- Salt

DIRECTIONS

1. Put the flour in a small bowl and the bread crumbs in a separate bowl.
2. Working with one chop at a time, lightly coat each in the flour, then dip in the beaten eggs and then in the bread crumbs. Gently press the bread crumbs into the pork chops so that much of the coating sticks.
3. Put ½ cup of clarified butter into a large skillet over medium-low heat. Working in two batches, heat the butter and add two chops. Cook on one side for 7 to 8 minutes, then flip and cook an additional 7 to 8 minutes until fully cooked. Add the remaining ½ cup of butter and repeat with the other two chops.
4. Serve immediately.

Meat

Spinach-stuffed Chicken Parmesan

Prep Time: 25 min
Cook Time: 30 min
Servings: 5

INGREDIENTS

- 4 cups fresh spinach
- 2 garlic cloves, minced
- 2 tsps. olive oil
- 2 tbsps. grated Parmesan cheese, divided
- 1/4 tsp. salt
- 1/4 tsp. pepper
- 4 boneless skinless chicken breast halves (4 oz. each)
- 1/2 cup dry whole wheat bread crumbs
- 1 large egg, lightly beaten
- 2 cans (8 oz. each) no-salt-added tomato sauce
- 1 tsp. dried basil
- 1 tsp. dried oregano
- 3/4 cup shredded part-skim mozzarella cheese

DIRECTIONS

1. Preheat the oven to 375 degrees. Cook and stir garlic and spinach in a big pan with oil until just wilted; drain. Mix in pepper, salt, and 1tsbp Parmesan cheese.
2. Use a meat mallet to lb. the chicken breast until a quarter-inch thick. Slather 1tsbp spinach mixture on each. Fold the chicken over the filling to enclose; use toothpicks to secure.
3. In separate shallow bowls, put egg and breadcrumbs. Submerge the chicken in egg then coat in crumbs. Arrange in an 8-inch cooking-spray-coated baking dish with the seam-side down. Bake for 20mins without cover.
4. In the meantime, mix oregano, basil, and tomato sauce in a big bowl; pour all over the chicken. Top with the remaining Parmesan cheese and mozzarella cheese. Bake for another 10-15mins without cover until a thermometer registers 165 degrees. Remove the toothpicks then serve.

NUTRITION: Calories: 281 Calories | Total Carbohydrate: 14 g | Cholesterol: 104 mg | Total Fat: 10 g | Fiber: 2 g | Protein: 31 g | Sodium: 432 mg

---

Rabbit Stew

Prep Time: 15 min
Cook Time: 1 hour
Servings: 4

INGREDIENTS

- ¼ cup pine nuts, lightly toasted
- ¼ teaspoon freshly grated nutmeg
- 1 pound mixed mushrooms, cut (cremini, button, shiitake, oyster, chanterelle, porcini)
- 2 cups dry white wine
- 2 tablespoons chopped fresh Italian parsley
- 2 teaspoons kosher salt
- 3 tablespoons extra-virgin olive oil
- 3 tablespoons tomato paste
- 4 sprigs fresh sage, tied with kitchen twine
- 4-pound rabbit, cut into 8 pieces
- 8 garlic cloves, crushed and peeled
- All-purpose flour, for dredging

DIRECTIONS

1. Flavour the rabbit with a of teaspoon salt. In a shallow basin, strew the flour and dredge the seasoned rabbit in it.
2. Heat the olive oil in a large Dutch oven over medium to high heat. Remove the rabbit pieces to a platter after searing them on all sides until well browned, about ten minutes.
3. Toss in the garlic cloves into the saucepan. Drop the tomato paste into a hot area and cook until it becomes slightly darker, about one minute, then stir until it is thoroughly combined with the garlic. Boil the white wine until it has been reduced by half, then add the nutmeg and sage.
4. Return the liquid to a rapid simmer after adding 2 cups hot water.
5. Once the liquid has reached a simmer, add the mushrooms and rabbit. Stir in the remaining salt and cover to keep it warm. Simmer until the rabbit is extremely soft, about 45 minutes, adding a little extra boiling water if necessary to keep the rabbit at least halfway covered.
6. Remove the garlic and sage sprigs from the rabbit before serving, and mix in the pine nuts and parsley.

Eggs and Sauce

Marinara Sauce

Prep Time 15 min   **Cook Time** 16 min   **Servings** 3 cups of sauce

- 1 (28 oz.) can San Marzano whole peeled tomatoes
- 1 large onion, diced
- 1 large carrot, diced
- 2 large cloves garlic, minced
- 1/4 cup olive oil
- 1 teaspoon basil, crushed
- 1/4 cup parsley
- 2 teaspoons salt, or to taste

1. Pour tomatoes into a bowl and crush with spoon or hands. In a medium saucepan, simmer tomatoes, onion and carrots for 15 minutes. Puree in blender and return to saucepan.
2. In a small skillet, sauté garlic in olive oil for 1 minute. Add to tomato mixture and cook 5 minutes more. Stir in basil, parsley and salt just before serving. Serve over cooked pasta.

Slim Italian Deviled Eggs

Prep Time 20 min   **Cook Time** 0 min   **Servings** 4

- 6 hard-boiled large eggs
- 3 tablespoons reduced-fat mayonnaise
- 1/4 teaspoon dried basil
- 1/4 teaspoon dried oregano
- 1/8 teaspoon salt
- 1/8 teaspoon pepper
- Shredded Parmesan cheese and fresh parsley, optional

1. Slice eggs in half lengthways. Scoop yolks out of eggs; put four yolks and whites aside (get rid of remaining yolks or reserve for another use).
2. Mash reserved yolks in a large bowl. Mix pepper, salt, oregano, basil, and mayonnaise in. Fill yolk mixture into egg whites. Use parsley and cheese for garnish if needed. Chilled till serving time.

Nutrition: Calories: 39 Cal | Protein: 3g | Total Fat: 3g | Sodium: 85mg | Fiber: 0 | Total Carbohydrate: 1g | Cholesterol: 70mg

Pasta Sauce with Italian Sausage

Prep Time 30 min   **Cook Time** 1 hour   **Servings** 6

- 1 pound Italian sausage links
- ½ pound lean ground beef
- 1 tablespoon olive oil
- 1 onion, chopped
- 1 clove garlic, chopped
- 1 (16 ounce) can canned tomatoes
- 1 (15 ounce) can canned tomato sauce
- 1 teaspoon salt
- ¼ teaspoon ground black pepper
- 1 teaspoon dried basil
- 1 teaspoon dried oregano
- 1 bay leaf

1. Removed casing from sausage links and cut into 1/2 inch slices. In a large skillet, brown sausage over medium heat for about 10 minutes; remove and set aside.
2. Sausage links' casings were removed and cut into 1/2-inch slices. Brown sausage for about 10 minutes in a large skillet over medium heat; remove and put aside.
3. Heat the ground beef, olive oil, garlic, and onion in a large skillet over medium heat until the meat is thoroughly browned; drain.
4. Mix in salt, black pepper, basil, oregano, bay leaf, and cooked sausage with tomatoes and tomato sauce. Cook, stirring periodically, for 1 hour, uncovered.
5. Bring a big saucepan of lightly salted water to a boil. Cook for 8 to 10 minutes, or until pasta is al dente; drain.
6. Before serving, combine the cooked sauce with the heated pasta and remove the bay leaf from the sauce.

NUTRITION: Calories: 339 Cal | Carbohydrate: 11.4 g | Fat: 24.6g | Protein: 18.5g | Sodium: 1547mg

Eggs and Sauces

Tuna Sauce

Prep Time 5 min   **Cook Time** 10 min   **Servings** 4

INGREDIENTS
- 400 g Peeled tomatoes
- 150 g Tuna in oil, drained
- 320 g Spaghetti
- ½ Golden onion
- Black pepper to taste
- Extra virgin olive oil to taste
- Salt to taste
- Basil to taste

DIRECTIONS
1. Start by bringing salted water to boil. You will use this water in cooking pasta. Meanwhile peel and chop the onion thinly. Add olive oil to a pan and fry the onion. Sauté for a few minutes while stirring until onions are dry.
2. Use your hands to fray the tuna and put it on the pan. Sauté for some minutes until it is brown as you stir occasionally. Use a fork to mash the tomatoes and then add to the pan. Cook for about 9-11 minutes.
3. At the meantime, boil the spaghetti and cook al dente. As the pasta cooks, the sauce will be ready. Drain straight into tuna pan.
4. Use pepper to season and then turn the heat off. Add basil leaves and mix the spaghetti and tuna and serve.

Italian Omelet

Prep Time 15 min   **Cook Time** 10 min   **Servings** 4

INGREDIENTS
- 1/2 cup chopped onions
- 2 cups of cholesterol-free egg product
- 4 oz. frozen ground turkey sausage, thawed

DIRECTIONS
1. Use cooking spray to coat a medium non-stick frying pan. Add sausage and onions; cook, and occasionally stir for 5 minutes or up to when sausage is browned on all sides.
2. Into a frying pan, pour the egg product; cook with a lid on for 5 minutes; pour the sausage mixture over.
3. Fold the omelet in half with the spatula; cover with the lid and cook for an additional 3 minutes.

Tomato Sauce

Prep Time 30 min   **Cook Time** 15 min   **Servings** 4

INGREDIENTS
- 3 tablespoons olive oil
- ½ small onion, finely diced
- 2 tablespoons chopped fresh parsley
- 2 or 3 garlic cloves, finely chopped
- 1 (28-ounce) can high-quality crushed tomatoes (see Choosing Quality Ingredients)
- 1 cup water
- ½ teaspoon salt
- 3 to 5 fresh basil leaves

DIRECTIONS
1. In a medium saucepan over medium-low heat, heat the oil for 1 minute. Add the onion and parsley. Once the onion is translucent, about 2 minutes, add the garlic and cook for 1 minute more.
2. Carefully add the tomatoes; they will splatter as they hit the hot oil. Add the water, salt, and basil leaves. Reduce the heat to low, cover, and let simmer for 20 minutes.

Tiramisu

Prep Time: 30 min
Cook Time: 15 min
Servings: 4

- 2 big pasteurized egg yolks
- 2 big pasteurized egg whites 10 tablespoon.
- (125 g) sugar.
- 1 cup (250 g) mascarpone.
- tsp. (25 ml) brandy (optional).
- 1 mug (200 ml) sweetened coffee.
- 8 savoiardi (girl fingers).
- bitter chocolate powder, as required

1. In a dish, beat eggs yolks with a lot of sugar, heating up mixture slightly in a heatproof bowl that fits comfortably over a pot of barely simmering water. in anvarious other bowl, blend egg whites with continuing to be sugar.
2. Mix mascarpone right into egg yolks, then include stiff egg whites and also thoroughly fold so mix remains light and frothy.
3. Dip lady fingers in sweetened coffee (if you wish you can include a little brandy) and also put them in all-time low of a dish (or in 4 small meals or glasses). then gather a layer of cream mixture as well as proceed rotating layers of biscuits and cream. Cool tiramisù For concerning 2 hours
4. Garnish with a generous sprinkling of chocolate.

Spinach Pasta Sauce

Prep Time: 25 min
Cook Time: 1 hour and 25 min
Servings: 10

- 1-1/2 lbs. Johnsonville® Ground Mild Italian sausage
- 3 cups sliced fresh mushrooms
- 1/2 cup each chopped carrot, green pepper and onion
- 1 can (28 oz.) crushed tomatoes
- 1 can (15 oz.) tomato sauce
- 1 can (6 oz.) tomato paste
- 1/2 cup grated Parmesan cheese
- 1/2 cup beef broth or red wine
- 3/4 tsp. each aniseed, seasoned salt, pepper, garlic powder, brown sugar, dried basil and oregano
- 4 cups coarsely chopped fresh spinach
- Hot cooked pasta
- 2 cups shredded mozzarella cheese
- 1/4 cup crumbled cooked bacon

1. Cook and crumble the sausage in a Dutch oven until it turns brown; drain. Add the carrot, mushrooms, onion and green pepper; sauté for about 5 minutes. Stir in the sauce, tomatoes, paste, broth, seasonings and Parmesan; make it to simmer for an hour while covered. Add the spinach and completely heat. Serve alongside the pasta; garnish with bacon and mozzarella.

NUTRITION: Calories 274 Cal | Fats 21 g | Sodium 1049 mg | Carbs 17 g | Protein 18 g | Cholesterol: 50 mg

Italian Cloud Eggs

Prep Time: 15 min
Cook Time: 25 min
Servings: 4

- 4 large eggs, separated
- 1/4 tsp. Italian seasoning
- 1/8 tsp. salt
- 1/8 tsp. pepper
- 1/4 cup shredded Parmesan cheese
- 1 tbsp. minced fresh basil
- 1 tbsp. finely chopped oil-packed sun-dried tomatoes

1. Set an oven to preheat to 450 degrees. Separate the eggs. In a big bowl, put the whites and place the yolks in another 4 small bowls. Beat the pepper, salt, Italian seasoning and egg whites until it forms stiff peaks.
2. Drop the egg white mixture into 4 mounds in a 9-inch cast iron skillet that was generously coated with cooking spray. Make a small well in the middle of each mound using the back of a spoon, then sprinkle cheese on top. Let it bake for around 5 minutes, until it becomes light brown. Slip an egg yolk gently into each of the mounds, then let it bake for another 3-5 minutes until the yolks become set. Sprinkle it with tomatoes and basil, then serve right away.

NUTRITION: Calories: 96 Cal | Carbohydrate: 1 g | Fat: 6 g | Fiber: 0 g | Protein: 8 g | Sodium: 234 mg

Eggs and Sauces

Mushroom Sausage Omelets

Prep Time 20 min
Cook Time 15 min
Servings 4

INGREDIENTS
- 1 fresh Johnsonville® Mild Italian Sausage Links (4-oz), casing removed
- 1-1/2 cups sliced fresh mushrooms
- 10 large eggs
- 1/2 cup grated Parmesan cheese
- 2 to 4 garlic cloves, minced
- 1/4 tsp. of pepper
- 1/4 - 1/2 cup of minced parsley
- 4 tsp. olive oil, divided

DIRECTIONS
1. Cook mushrooms and sausage in a 10-in. nonstick frying pan over medium-high heat, until the sausage is no pinker, about 4-6 minutes, crushing the sausage into small pieces. Use a slotted spoon to take out; clean the frying pan.
2. Combine pepper, garlic, cheese, and eggs in a big bowl until combined. Mix in parsley.
3. Heat 2 tsp. Of oil in the same frying pan over medium-high heat. Add half of the egg mixture. The edges of the mixture should set immediately. While the eggs are set, let the raw eggs run underneath and push the cooked eggs toward the middle. Once the eggs are hardened, and no liquid egg left, put on one side with half of the sausage mixture; fold omelet in half.
4. Slice the omelet into two; put on serving dishes—Cook the rest of the ingredients in the same way.

Oven-Baked Eggs and Asparagus

Prep Time 15 min
Cook Time 20 min
Servings 2

- 2 tsp. of olive oil
- ½ of a large onion, cut thinly
- 1 bundle of asparagus, trimmed and cut into chunks
- Salt and pepper to taste
- 10 eggs, beaten
- ¾ cup parmesan cheese, grated

1. In a pan, heat the oil and sauté the onions.
2. Add the asparagus and sauté until it is crispy. Season it with pepper and salt, and then set aside.
3. Grease the plate and divide vegetables and the eggs between them.
4. Top with the parmesan cheese.
5. Then, preheated oven to 380 degrees F. Bake for about 30 minutes or until the cheese at the top turns brown.

Crockpot Pasta Sauce With Meat

Prep Time 15 min
Cook Time 10-12 hours
Servings 4 quarts of sauce

- 2 lb. lean ground beef
- 2 yellow onions, chopped
- 3 cloves garlic, crushed
- 5 (28 oz. each) cans San Marzano whole peeled tomatoes, well drained
- 1 (16 oz.) can tomato paste
- 2 (8 oz.) cans tomato sauce
- 2 teaspoons dried basil
- 2 teaspoons dried oregano
- 2 teaspoons granulated sugar
- 2 teaspoons salt
- 1 teaspoon pepper

DIRECTIONS
1. In a large skillet, brown ground beef with onions and garlic. Place in a 5 to 6-quart crockpot. Put well drained tomatoes in blender or food processor and puree until smooth. Add to crockpot. Add remaining ingredients and stir well. Cook in crockpot 10 to 12 hours on low heat.

Arrabbiata Sauce

Prep Time 15 min

Cook Time 10 min

Servings 4

INGREDIENTS

- 380 g Peeled tomatoes, dried
- 3 dry small chilies
- 1 Garlic clove
- Extra virgin olive oil to taste
- Parsley to taste
- 320 g Penne Rigate
- Salt to taste

DIRECTIONS

1. In preparation of Arrabbiata sauce, begin with draining the peeled tomatoes. After that, transfer them in a bowl and use a fork to mash and then chop them.
2. At this given point, use a knife to chop the dried chili and use your hands to crumble it. On the fire, put a pan filled with water add salt to taste and then cook the pasta.
3. In a pan, pour in a generous oil amount and add the chili pepper and peeled garlic clove. Leave then gently and then add tomatoes and then mix everything together then use salt to season. Cook for about 12 minutes while they are covered with a lid and occasionally stir.
4. Cook the pasta al dente by following the cooking times that are shown on the package when the sauce is almost cooked. Remove the lid and remove the garlic after 12 minutes. Drain the pasta and directly transfer it to the sauce.
5. For a moment, skip it and if necessary, add the cooking water. Add chopped parsley and mix for one more and last time and then you can serve your sauce.

STORAGE
It's advisable to consume the Arrabbiata sauce while it is still fresh. As an alternative, you can keep in the refrigerator for 1 day.

ADVICE
Garnish each dish using pecorino Romana and also use fresh chili.

Old Italian Meat Sauce

Prep Time 30 min

Cook Time 4 hours

Servings 20

- 2 pounds lean ground beef
- 1 pound ground pork
- 2 tablespoons olive oil
- 2 medium (2-1/2" dia)s onions, chopped
- 1 clove garlic, crushed
- 3 cups red wine
- 2 pounds fresh mushrooms, sliced
- ¼ teaspoon dried rosemary
- 4 tablespoons chopped fresh oregano
- ¼ teaspoon chopped fresh thyme
- 3 (29 ounce) cans tomato sauce
- 1 (6 ounce) can tomato paste
- 2 tablespoons grated Parmesan cheese

1. In a large skillet, brown the meat and pork over medium heat until no longer pink; put aside.
2. Warm olive oil in a large skillet over medium heat and cook onions and garlic until soft; add about 1/2 cup wine and stir thoroughly.
3. Add another 1/2 cup wine to the skillet and cook the mushrooms, rosemary, oregano, and thyme until soft.
4. Toss in the browned meat, tomato sauce, and tomato paste; cook for 1 hour before adding the remaining 2 cups of wine.

NUTRITION: Calories: 260 Cal | Carbohydrate: 15.9g | Fat: 16.8g | Protein: 15.3g | Sodium: 788mg

Eggs and Sauces

Puttanesca Sauce

Prep Time 20 min **Cook Time** 20 min **Servings** 4

INGREDIENTS
- 10 g Capers in salt
- 800 g Peeled tomatoes
- 3 Garlic cloves
- 1 bunch Parsley to be minced
- 30 g Extra virgin olive oil
- 320 g Spaghetti
- 25 g Anchovies in oil
- 2 Dry chilies
- 100 g Gaeta olives
- Salt to taste

DIRECTIONS
1. To make the puttanesca sauce, begin with rinsing the capers under running water in order to remove the excess salt. Dry them and put them on a cutting board to coarsely chop them.
2. Use the knife blade to mash the pitted Gaeta olives. Also wash the parsley, dry it and then mince it.
3. On the fire, put a full pot of water and bring it to boil, once it boils, add salt. This water will be used for pasta cooking.
4. In a large pan, pour the chopped dried chilies, peeled and left garlic cloves and oil. Add the desalted capers and anchovy fillets.
5. Over medium heat, brown them for at least 5 minutes while you are stirring occasionally so that the anchovies release all the aromas after melting.
6. Pour the lightly crushed and peeled tomatoes at this point and use a spoon to mix and then over medium heat, cook them for another 10 minutes. In the meantime, boil the spaghetti al dente.
7. Remove the garlic cloves and add the crushed olives once the sauce is ready. Use chopped fresh parsley to flavor the sauce.
8. Meanwhile bring the pasta to cooking and then directly drain it in a pan and then sauté for half a minute. This time is enough to mix all flavors.
9. You may now serve the puttanesca sauce still hot.

STORAGE
It's not recommended to freeze.
It's advisable to consume the spaghetti puttanesca immediately. You can cover them using a plastic wrap and keep them in the refrigerator for 1 day if they advance.

ADVICE
You can make a fresh and good sauce when the tomatoes are in season.
We recommend you to avoid adding more salt since this dish is very savory.

Fettuccine Sauce

Prep Time 25 min **Cook Time** 15 min **Servings** 5

INGREDIENTS
- 6 oz. uncooked fettuccine
- 2 tbsp. minced fresh basil
- 1 small green pepper, chopped
- 1 small onion, chopped
- 1 tbsp. olive oil
- 1 can (15-oz) of black beans
- 1 tsp. dried oregano
- 2 cups garden-style pasta sauce
- 1/2 tsp. fennel seed
- 1/4 tsp. garlic salt
- 1 cup shredded part-skim mozzarella cheese

DIRECTIONS
1. Cook the fettuccine following the package instructions. In the meantime, sauté onion and green pepper in a big saucepan with oil until tender. Mix in seasonings, black beans, and pasta sauce.
2. Boil, then lower the heat. Let it simmer for 5mins without a cover. Drain the fettuccine. Add sauce and sprinkled cheese on top.

Pesto Sauce

Prep Time 20 min | **Cook Time** 30 min | **Servings** 2

INGREDIENTS

- 50 ml Extra virgin olive oil
- 15 g Grated Pecorino
- 25 g Basil leaves
- 35 g Parmesan cheese DOP to be grated
- 1 pinch coarse salt.
- 8 g Pine nuts
- ½ Garlic clove

DIRECTIONS

1. In preparing the pesto sauce, make sure you specify that basil leaves shouldn't be washed but you only use a soft cloth to clean them. You as well ensure that Genoese or Ligurian basil that has leaves that are narrow.
2. To prepare the pesto, put together coarse salt and some peeled garlic in a mortar. Start crushing and once the garlic reduces to cream, add a pinch of coarse salt and basil leaves together and these will help in crushing the fibers better and also help in maintaining the bright and beautiful green color.
3. Against the walls of the mortar, crush the basil by turning the mortar in the opposite direction simultaneously and also turning the pestle from left to right taking it y its ears. Continue doing this until you get a bright and green liquid from the basil leaves. At this particular point, to reduce to cream, add pine nuts and begin beating again.
4. Constantly stir after adding cheese, little at a given time to make the sauce creamier and add extra virgin olive oil as the last one and use a pestle to mix after pouring it flush.
5. Mix all ingredients until you get a homogeneous sauce. The Genoese pesto is now ready for you to use.

Crockpot Pasta Sauce With Meat

Prep Time 15 min | **Cook Time** 10-12 hours | **Servings** 4 quarts of sauce

INGREDIENTS

- 2 lb. lean ground beef
- 2 yellow onions, chopped
- 3 cloves garlic, crushed
- 5 (28 oz. each) cans San Marzano whole peeled tomatoes, well drained
- 1 (16 oz.) can tomato paste
- 2 (8 oz.) cans tomato sauce
- 2 teaspoons dried basil
- 2 teaspoons dried oregano
- 2 teaspoons granulated sugar
- 2 teaspoons salt
- 1 teaspoon pepper

DIRECTIONS

1. In a large skillet, brown ground beef with onions and garlic. Place in a 5 to 6-quart crockpot. Put well drained tomatoes in blender or food processor and puree until smooth. Add to crockpot. Add remaining ingredients and stir well. Cook in crockpot 10 to 12 hours on low heat.

Eggs and Sauces

Italian Basil Baked Eggs

Prep Time 10 min | **Cook Time** 20 min | **Servings** 7

- ½ teaspoon salt
- ½ cup basil
- 2 garlic cloves
- 7 eggs
- ½ teaspoon thyme
- 7 teaspoon olive oil
- 7 oz Cheddar cheese
- 1 cup cherry tomatoes

1. Grate Cheddar cheese.
2. Wash the basil and chop it.
3. Slice the cherry tomatoes and garlic cloves.
4. After this, sprinkle the cast-iron pan with the olive oil and preheat it.
5. Add the cherry tomatoes and garlic cloves and simmer the mixture for 5 minutes on the medium heat.
6. Then sprinkle it with the basil and thyme.
7. Cook the vegetables for 2 minutes more.
8. After this, preheat the oven to 360 F.
9. Crack the eggs into the vegetable mixture.
10. Sprinkle the eggs with the salt and grated Cheddar cheese.
11. Put the dish in the preheated oven and cook it for 10 minutes more.
12. When the eggs are baked – remove them from the oven and chill well.
13. Serve the cooked dish warm.

NUTRITION: Calories 22 | Fat 16.7g | Fiber 0 | Carbohydrates 4.58g | Protein 13g

---

Pizza Sauce

Prep Time 5 min | **Cook Time** 0 | **Servings** 24

- 1 (15 ounce) can tomato sauce
- 1 1/2 teaspoons dried minced garlic
- 1 (6 ounce) can tomato paste
- 1 teaspoon ground paprika
- 1 tablespoon ground oregano

1. In a medium bowl, Mix together tomato sauce and tomato paste until smooth. Stir in oregano, garlic and paprika

NUTRITION: Calories: 11Cal | Carbs: 2.6g | Fat: 0.1g | Protein: 0.6g | Cholesterol: 0mg

---

Italian Egg Toast

Prep Time 25 min | **Cook Time** 10 min | **Servings** 2

INGREDIENTS

- ½ cup of pizza sauce
- 2 slices of bread
- 2 eggs
- 1 ½ tbsp. of olive oil
- 4 tbsp. of shredded mozzarella cheese
- Some Italian seasonings

DIRECTIONS

1. Heat the pizza sauce in a skillet and set aside.
2. Heat the oil in a skillet, crack in the eggs and cook until the whites are set.
3. Toast the bread slices, divide the pizza sauce, cheese, and eggs on each toast

Scented Deviled Eggs

Prep Time: 10 min | **Cook Time:** 0 min | **Servings:** 8

INGREDIENTS
- 8 eggs, boiled
- 3 tablespoon Romano cheese
- 1 teaspoon paprika
- 2 tablespoon pesto sauce
- 1 tablespoon mayo sauce
- 1 teaspoon mustard
- ½ teaspoon ground black pepper
- 1 tablespoon dill
- 1 teaspoon lime juice

DIRECTIONS
1. Peel the eggs and cut them into the halves.
2. Then remove the egg yolks from the eggs and mash them carefully in the separated bowl with the help of the fork.
3. After this, add the mustard, mayo sauce, pesto sauce, and lime juice.
4. Blend the mixture with the help of the hand blender.
5. Then season the smooth mixture with the ground black pepper and paprika.
6. Add dill.
7. Grate Romano cheese and add it to the egg yolk mixture too.
8. Stir it carefully with the fork again.
9. Then fill the pastry bag with the egg yolk mixture and fill the egg whites with it.
10. Put the cooked eggs in the fridge and keep them there till you serve them.

NUTRITION: Calories 157 Cal | Fat 12g | Fiber 0 | Carbs 2.29g | Protein 10g

---

Italian Meat Sauce

Prep Time: 45 min | **Cook Time:** 5 hours | **Servings:** 12

INGREDIENTS
- 1/4 cup olive oil
- 1 onion, chopped
- 6 garlic cloves, sliced
- 3 15oz-can seasoned tomato sauce
- 3 14.5oz-cans diced tomatoes with juice
- 6 cups water
- 8 6oz-cans tomato paste
- 2 pounds Italian sausage
- 2 pounds ground sirloin
- 4 tablespoons chopped fresh parsley
- 1 cup grated Romano cheese
- 2 tbsp. dried oregano
- salt and pepper to taste
- 1 pound pork meat, cubed
- 1 cup dry bread crumbs
- 3 tablespoons garlic powder
- 1/3 cup grated Parmesan cheese
- 2 large eggs

DIRECTIONS
1. In large pot heat 2 tablespoons olive oil over low heat. Combine the chopped onion and two-thirds of the sliced garlic in a mixing bowl. 5 minutes of sautéing Tomato sauce, diced tomatoes, water, and tomato paste are added to the pan. Simmer.
2. Meanwhile, heat the remaining olive oil in a large skillet over medium heat. Cook for another 1 to 2 minutes with the remaining garlic. Brown the sausage for three minutes on each side. Cover and lower heat after browning. Cook for 10 minutes, then remove the sausages from the heat and cut them in half. Toss with the tomato mixture.
3. In a sausage skillet, cook the pork over medium heat. Toss with the tomato mixture. To the tomato sauce, add 3 tablespoons parsley, Romano, oregano, salt, and pepper. Continue to cook on a low heat setting.
4. Preheat the oven to 375 degrees Fahrenheit (190 degrees C). Aluminum foil should be used to cover a cookie sheet. Combine garlic powder, ground sirloin, bread crumbs, garlic powder, remaining parsley, parmesan, and eggs in a large mixing basin. Form into one-inch balls and placed on a cookie sheet. Cook for about 20 minutes, or until golden brown. Toss the meatballs into the sauce. Cook the sauce for another 5 hours. Serve with fusilli or ravioli as a side dish.

NUTRITION: Calories 660 Cal | Fat 35.5g | Sodium 2451mg | Carbohydrates 46g | Protein 42g

Eggs and Sauces

Tomato and Basil Sauce

Prep Time 10 min **Cook Time** 30 min **Servings** 6

- 700 ml Tomato sauce
- 400 g Tomato pulp
- ½ onion
- Salt to taste
- 1 pinch of sugar
- Fresh basil leaves

1. In making the tomato sauce quickly, begin by chopping the golden or the white onion.
2. Put a pot on the oven and put the onions that you chopped and allow then to get soft very well. To avoid darkening, make sure you turn it often.
3. Add the tomato puree and use salt and a pinch of sugar to season it because this helps to reduce the tomato acidity and also add the tomato pulp in small pieces. Allow the sauce to boil over medium heat while its covered.
4. Low the heat once it begins boiling and allow it to cook for 20-25 minutes. Season the sauce with fresh basil leaves that are finely chopped.
5. The tomato sauce is now ready to be used as you like it.

Italian Pesto Hollandaise

Prep Time 45 min **Cook Time** 10 min **Servings** 4

- 1 tbsp. prepared pesto
- 4 slices Italian bread (1 inch thick), toasted
- 4 large egg yolks
- 2 tbsp. water
- 1 tbsp. lemon juice
- 2 tsp. white vinegar
- 4 large eggs
- 1/2 cup butter, cubed
- 8 thin slices of prosciutto or deli ham
- 4 fresh basil leaves
- 4 slices tomato

1. Melt butter in a small pot; mix in pesto. Whisk lemon juice, water, and egg yolks in a metal bowl cook while constantly mixing until it reaches 160 degrees and is thick enough to cover a metal spoon. Turn to very low heat; pour in warm melted butter mixture very slowly while constantly mixing.
2. Move to a small bowl, then set the bowl in a giant bowl with warm water. Mix from time to time while keeping warm until serving. Pour 2 to 3 inches of water in a big pot or pan with high sides; pour in vinegar, then boil. Adjust heat to keep a gentle simmer. Break one cold egg in a small bowl; keep the bowl close over the water, then slide each egg in the water.
3. Cook for 3-5mins without cover until the yolks start to thicken yet not complicated and the whites are set completely. Lift the eggs out with a slotted spoon.
4. On a toast, layer tomato, basil, prosciutto, and eggs. Add hollandaise sauce on top, then serve right away.

Clam Sauce

Prep Time 20 min **Cook Time** 20 min **Servings** 4

- 1 bunch Parsley
- 1 kg Clams
- 320 g Spaghetti
- 1 clove Garlic
- Coarse salt for clams to taste
- Salt to taste
- Black pepper to taste
- Extra virgin olive oil to taste

1. Clean the spaghetti and discard any broken shells. Break them on a cutting board or beat them against a sink. This helps in checking if there is sand present inside; the bivalves without sand will be closed while the ones with sand will open. Put a colander in a bowl and place the clams inside to rinse them. Put colander in a bowl and sprinkle with lots of salt. Let the clams soak for about two and half hours.
2. After that tie, any residual sand will be purged. Heat oil in saucepan under medium heat and add garlic. Carefully drain the clams, rinse and immerse them in the pan. Cover and cook on high heat for several minutes.
3. When heated, the clams will open. Occasionally shake the pan as you cook until they open fully. Turn the heat off when they all open. Drain the bivalves and collect the juice. Meanwhile, add the spaghetti to boiling salted water and when you are halfway through, drain them.
4. Pour sauce into a pan. Pour the spaghetti in too and go on cooking. When done with cooking, add chopped parsley and the clams and blast once and your meal is ready.
5. Serve and enjoy immediately.

Italian Red Sauce

Prep Time: 10 min
Cook Time: 2 hours and 10 min
Servings: 12

- 3 chopped roma (plum) tomatoes
- 12 onion, finely chopped
- 1 can sliced black olives, 2.25 oz., drained
- 1 drained and chopped 6 oz. marinated artichoke heart
- 2 tablespoons lemon jucei
- 1 tsp garlic, minced
- 3 tbsp. chopped basil leaves
- 14 teaspoon red pepper flakes, crushed
- 14 teaspoon seasoning (Italian)
- 14 teaspoon cumin powder
- 3 tblsp fresh cilantro, chopped
- a quarter teaspoon of salt
- 1/8 teaspoon black pepper, ground

1. In a bowl, gently combine the tomatoes, onion, olives, and artichoke hearts; set aside. In a separate bowl, combine the garlic, lemon juice, basil, red pepper flakes, Italian seasoning, cumin, cilantro, salt, and pepper. Toss the tomato mixture with the dressing

NUTRITION: Calories 150 Cal | Fat 9.2g | Sodium 644mg | Carbohydrates 14g | Protein 3.1g

---

Baked Eggs & Sausage

Prep Time: 15 min
Cook Time: 30 min
Servings: 8

- 1 lb. Johnsonville® Ground Mild Italian sausage
- 1 jar (24 oz.) fire-roasted tomato and garlic pasta sauce
- 1 can (14-1/2 oz.) fire-roasted diced tomatoes, drained
- 3/4 cup part-skim ricotta cheese
- 8 large eggs
- 1/4 tsp. salt
- 1/4 tsp. pepper
- 1/4 cup shredded Parmesan cheese
- 1 tbsp. minced fresh basil
- 1 French bread demi-baguette (4 oz.), cut into 1-inch slices
- 1/4 cup butter, softened

1. Set an oven to 350 degrees and start preheating. Cook the sausage, crumbling the meat in a large skillet over medium heat until not pink anymore; then drain. Stir in tomatoes and pasta sauce. Arrange on a 13x9-inch baking dish.
2. Top the meat mixture with a dollop of ricotta cheese. Carefully break an egg in a small bowl; slip the egg onto ricotta. Repeat the process for the remaining eggs. Dust with Parmesan cheese, pepper, and salt.
3. Bake until the yolks start to become thick but not hard and the whites are set completely, 30-35 minutes. Take out of the oven and dust with basil.
4. At the same time, spread the butter over the bread slices; arrange them on an ungreased baking sheet. Preheat the broiler. Broil 3-4 inches from the heat source for 1-2 minutes per side until golden brown. Serve right away together with baked eggs.

NUTRITION: Calories: 408 Calories | Total Carbs: 22 g | Cholesterol: 241 mg | Total Fat: 27 g | Fiber: 3 g | Protein: 19 g | Sodium: 1183 mg

---

Mexican-Italian Salsa

Prep Time: 25 min
Cook Time: 0
Servings: 10

- 3 chopped roma (plum) tomatoes
- 12 onion, finely chopped
- 1 can sliced black olives, 2.25 oz., drained
- 1 drained and chopped 6 oz. marinated artichoke heart
- 2 tablespoons lemon jucei
- 1 tsp garlic, minced
- 3 tblsp basil leaves, chopped
- 1/4 teaspoon red pepper flakes, crushed
- 1/4 teaspoon seasoning (Italian)
- 1/4 teaspoon cumin powder
- 3 tblsp fresh cilantro, chopped
- a quarter teaspoon of salt
- 1/8 teaspoon black pepper, ground

1. In a bowl, gently combine the tomatoes, onion, olives, and artichoke hearts; set aside. In another bowl, combine the lemon juice, garlic, basil, red pepper flakes, Italian seasoning, cumin, cilantro, salt, and pepper. Toss the tomato mixture with the dressing.

NUTRITION: Calories: 31 Cal | Carbohydrate: 4.1 g | Fat: 1.7 g | Protein: 1 g | Sodium: 179mg

Eggs and Sauces

Italian Spaghetti Sauce with Meatballs

Prep Time 20 min **Cook Time** 2 hours and 20 min **Servings** 4

INGREDIENTS

Meatballs
- 1 pound lean ground beef
- 1 cup fresh bread crumbs
- 1 tablespoon dried parsley
- 1 tablespoon grated Parmesan cheese
- ¼ teaspoon ground black pepper
- ⅛ teaspoon garlic powder
- 1 egg, beaten

Sauce
- ¾ cup chopped onion
- 5 cloves garlic, minced
- ¼ cup olive oil
- 2 (28 ounce) cans whole peeled tomatoes
- 2 teaspoons salt
- 1 teaspoon white sugar
- 1 bay leaf
- 1 (6 ounce) can tomato paste
- ¾ teaspoon dried basil
- ½ teaspoon ground black pepper

1. Combine the ground, bread crumbs, parsley, Parmesan, black pepper, garlic powder, and egg in a large mixing bowl to create a mix for meatballs. A total of 15 balls can be made from this one. Cover and refrigerate the rolled meatball until ready to use.
2. Sauté the garlics and onion in olive oil over medium heat until onion is transparent. Combine the tomatoes, salt, sugar, and bay leaf in a mixing bowl. Cover, turn to low heat, and cook for 90 minutes. Cook for another 30 minutes after adding the tomato paste, basil, 1/2 teaspoon pepper, and meatballs. Serve.

Nutrition: Calories 346 Cal | Fat 21.2g | Sodium 1492mg | Carbohydrates 23g | Protein 19g

---

Italian Egg Bake

Prep Time 20 min **Cook Time** 1 hour and 5 min **Servings** 6

INGREDIENTS
- 4 slices sandwich bread, cubed
- 1/4 cup coarsely chopped fresh basil
- 1/4 cup soft sun-dried tomato halves (not packed in oil), finely chopped
- 6 bacon strips, cooked and crumbled
- 1 cup shredded part-skim mozzarella cheese
- 6 large eggs
- 2/3 cup 2% milk
- 1 garlic clove, minced
- 1/2 tsp. salt
- 1/4 tsp. pepper
- 1 tbsp. minced chives

DIRECTIONS

1. Layer 1/2 each of bread, basil, tomatoes, bacon and cheese in a greased 8-in. square baking dish. Repeat layers.
2. Beat pepper, salt, garlic, milk and eggs in a small bowl. Place over the layers. Cover and refrigerate for several hours or overnight.
3. Turn the oven to 350° and start preheating. Take casserole out of the fridge while oven heats. Bake with a cover for 30 minutes. Bake without a cover for another 15-20 minutes or until golden, puffed and the inserted knife in the center comes out clean. Dust with chives. Allow to sit for 5-10 minutes before cutting.

Porcini Mushrooms Sauce

Prep Time: 50 min
Cook Time: 15 min
Servings: 4

INGREDIENTS

For pasta
- Semolina to sprinkle to taste
- 120 g Fresh eggs
- 200 g 00 flour
- For seasoning
- 50 g Butter
- 500 g Porcini mushrooms
- Salt to taste
- 1 Garlic clove
- 1 Parsley sprig
- 35 g Extra virgin olive oil
- Black pepper to taste

DIRECTIONS

1. In preparation of Porcini mushrooms sauce, begin with the fresh pasta. In a bowl or pastry board, pour the flour, form a classic fountain shape and in the center, pour in the previously beaten eggs.
2. To get consistent dough that is not too dry or too sticky, it is advisable to respect the recommended egg doses. Using a fork, start mixing from the center and collect the flour gradually. Work with your hands and vigorously knead when the dough is more compact. Do this for about 10 minutes.
3. Give a spherical shape to the dough and use a cling film to wrap it and allow it to rest away from heat sources in a cool place at room temperature for 30 minutes.
4. In the meantime, concentrate on the porcini mushrooms. Using a small knife, scrap the stem and clean them from the soil. You can use a slightly dampened cloth to clean them if they are very dirty. You can as well pass them under cold running water quickly and then use a cloth to dry them perfectly. Mushrooms absorb too much water and so may lose their consistency and flavor so if you decide to use this option, do it so quickly and then cut them in slices.
5. On very low heat, pour the butter in a large saucepan and pour in the oil when the butter is almost melted completely. Allow it to slightly warm up and then pour in 1 whole garlic clove, you can chop it if you want and the porcini mushrooms.
6. Add pepper and salt to your taste and then cook the mushrooms for a period of 10 minutes. You can remove the whole garlic if you had added it after the cooking and once it is ready, keep it warm. Finely chop the parsley and set it aside.
7. Take the dough and divide it in 16 pieces after the necessary resting time. For the piece to be passed in the machine to be rolled, flour it lightly. Cover the remaining dough with a plastic wrap and keep it aside.
8. Passing from the largest to the penultimate thickness, insert the first piece into the machine and keep the remaining dough aside. Use a plastic wrap to cover it.
9. Once you reach to the penultimate step of the machine, Go again over the dough strip. To pull the dough well, two steps at this thickness will be required.
10. Use semolina flour to lightly flour the work surface and roll out the first sheet. Continue with the rest of the dough pieces until you make various sheets and sprinkle the sheets with semolina and allow them to dry for 5 minutes in order to finish the dough.
11. Of each sheet, fold the shorter side inwards and then roll the dough on itself. Begin making the tagliatelle by cutting to a 6.5-7 mm thickness using a lightly floured and sharp knife.
12. To make the nests of noodles, lift every roll and place them gradually on a tray or a work surface part that has been lightly floured with semolina flour.
13. Boil the water then add salt. Cook the noodles for 3-4 minutes. Directly drain into the seasoning. Keep the cooking water. On low heat, add the seasonings and ingredients in a pan and mix them together. Add the chopped parsley and to prevent the noodles from becoming too dry, you can add a ladle of pasta cooking water.
14. Now your noodles with porcini mushrooms are now ready. Serve and enjoy.

Eggs and Sauces

Classic Bolognese Sauce

Prep Time: 25 min
Cook Time: 4 hours and 15 min
Servings: 3 quarts

- 1/3 cup garlic cloves (about 6 fat cloves)
- ½ teaspoon kosher salt, plus more to taste
- 1 carrot, peeled and shredded
- 2 big celery stalks, minced in a food processor or finely chopped
- 2 cups canned Italian plum tomatoes, preferably San Marzano, and juices, passed through a food mill or crushed using your hands
- 2 cups dry red wine
- 2 cups dry white wine
- 2 medium onions, minced in a food processor or finely chopped
- 2 pounds ground beef
- 2 pounds ground pork
- 2 tablespoons extra-virgin olive oil
- 2 tablespoons tomato paste
- 6 ounces bacon or pancetta
- 8 to 12 cups (or more) hot Chicken Stock, Vegetable Stock, or plain hot water
- Freshly ground black pepper to taste

1. In a large mixing bowl, combine all ground meat in the ingredient. Crush and loosen everything using your fingertips, then mix and crumble the beef and pork together. Pour the wine over the meat and massage it between your fingers again to moisten it evenly.
2. To create the pestata, chop the bacon or pancetta into 1-inch pieces and combine with the garlic in the bowl of a food processor. Process them until they form a fine paste.
3. Scrape all of the pestata into a large Dutch oven with the olive oil. Set the pan over medium-high heat, break up the pestata, and stir it about the bottom of the pan to begin rendering the fat. Cook for 3-4 minutes, or until the fat has rendered.
4. Mix the minced onions into the fat, and cook for about 2 minutes, until sizzling and beginning to sweat. Mix in the celery and carrot, and cook until the vegetables are wilted and golden, stirring regularly and meticulously, on moderate to high heat, approximately five minutes or more.
5. Increase the heat, push the vegetables off to the side, and plop all the meat into the pan; drizzle the salt on. Give the meat on the pan bottom a little time to brown, then stir, spread, and toss with a sturdy spoon, mixing the meat into the vegetables and ensuring every bit of meat browns and starts releasing fat and juices. Soon the meat liquid will nearly cover the meat itself. Cook at high heat while stirring frequently, until all that liquid has disappeared, even in the bottom of the pan, approximately thirty to forty-five minutes, depending on the heat and the width of the pan. Stir once in a while, and as the liquid level lessens, reduce the heat so the meat doesn't burn.
6. Warm the broth in a moderate-sized deep cooking pan.
7. When all the meat liquid has been cooked off, pour in the red wine. Cook until the wine has nearly fully vaporized, approximately five minutes. Put in the tomato paste into a clear space on the pan bottom. Toast one minute in the hot spot, then stir to combine it with the meat, and allow it to caramelize for two or three minutes. Mix in the crushed tomatoes; slosh the tomato bowl out with a cup of hot broth and put in that. Bring the liquid to its boiling point, stirring the meat, and allow the liquid to nearly boil off off, five minutes more.
8. Pour in 2 cups of hot broth, stir thoroughly, and put in more if required to cover the meat. Bring it to a lively simmer, cover the pan, and regulate the heat to maintain slow, steady cooking, with small bubbles perking all on the surface of the sauce. From this point, the Bolognese should cook for an additional three hours. Check the pot every twenty minutes and put in hot broth as required to cover the meat. The liquid level must be reducing by 1½ to 2 cups between additions. Regulate the heat if the sauce is reducing faster than that or not as fast. Stir frequently to ensure the bottom doesn't burn.
9. Finally, you want to reduce the level of the liquid. When you're done, the meat should no longer be immersed but seem suspended in a dense, flowing liquid. If the meat is still submerged in a lot of liquid, remove the cover completely to cook off moisture swiftly. A few minutes before the end of cooking, taste a bit of meat and sauce, and put in salt if you wish. Grind 1 teaspoon of black pepper right into the sauce, stir it in, and cook about five minutes before you take the pan off the heat. If you'll be using the sauce immediately, spoon off the fat from the surface, or stir it in, as is done conventionally. Otherwise, allow the sauce to cool, then chill it meticulously and lift off the coagulated fat. Store the sauce for quite a few days in your fridge, or freeze it for use within a few months.

Snacks and Appetizers

Baked Pumpkin Flowers with Ricotta

Prep Time 15 min | **Cook Time** 10 min | **Servings** 2

INGREDIENTS
- 10 fresh pumpkin flowers
- 17.6 oz ricotta cheese
- 1 tablespoon grated Parmesan cheese
- 1 egg
- 2 leaves of fresh mint
- 1 pinch of salt
- 1 pinch of pepper
- 0.5 oz extra virgin olive oil

DIRECTIONS
1. Clean the squash blossoms, removing the pistil inside, then place them in a non-stick baking dish.
2. In a bowl, mix the ricotta, egg, grated Parmesan, salt, pepper and mint.
3. Gently fill the flowers with the help of a teaspoon, drizzle with a little oil and bake at 356°F for about 10 minutes.

NUTRITION: Calories: 107.2 Kcal | Carbs: 5.5 g | Protein: 10.1 g | Fat: 5.2 g | Fiber: 1.0 g

Amaretto Biscotti

Prep Time 15 min | **Cook Time** 40 min | **Servings** 4-5 dozen

INGREDIENTS
- 1/2 cup butter
- 1 1/2 cups granulated sugar
- 3 eggs
- 1 teaspoon Amaretto liqueur
- 1 tablespoon anise seed
- 1 teaspoon lemon rind, grated
- 1 cup walnuts, chopped
- 3 cups all-purpose flour
- 3 teaspoons baking powder
- 1/2 teaspoon salt

DIRECTIONS
1. Preheat oven to 350 degrees F. In a large bowl, cream butter and sugar. Add beaten eggs, Amaretto, anise seed, lemon rind and walnuts. Add flour, which has been mixed with baking powder and salt.
2. Knead into a roll, adding more flour to the surface so it won't stick. Cut into 5 rolls and shape into flattened loaves. Place on a greased cookie sheet. Bake at 350 degrees F. 25 to 30 minutes. Cool slightly; cut diagonally and return to oven for an additional 10 minutes.

Canapes with avocado cream

Prep Time: 30 min
Cook Time: 10 min
Servings: 20 pieces

INGREDIENTS

- 10 quail eggs
- 10 slices of roast turkey rump without skin
- 6 slices of bread
- 1 spring onion
- 7 oz diced avocado
- ½ pot of unsweetened white yogurt
- 1.4 oz extra virgin olive oil
- 1 oz lemon juice
- 2 pinches of salt
- 2 grinds of pepper

DIRECTIONS

1. Turn on the oven to 356°F.
2. Place the quail eggs in cold water and bring to a boil. Cook for 5 minutes. Then run them under cold water.
3. Place the turkey in a bowl and season with 0.6 oz oil, 0.5 oz lemon juice, 1 pinch salt, 1 pinch pepper and the spring onion cut into rings. Cover with plastic wrap and store in the refrigerator.
4. Peel the eggs.
5. Cut the bread into 2-inch squares on each side and toast for 5-10 minutes in the oven.
6. In a food processor, place the avocado, yogurt, remaining lemon juice, remaining oil, 1 pinch salt, 1 pinch pepper and blend.
7. Transfer the mixture to a pastry bag.
8. Remove the turkey rump from the fridge and let it drain well from the marinade, then cut the slices in half.
9. Stuff each tartlet with the avocado cream, turkey rump, half an egg and the spring onion rings.
10. Serve.

NUTRITION: Calories: 62.5 cal. | Carbs: 3.4 g. | Protein: 2.9 g. | Fat: 4.5 g. | Fiber: 0.8 g

---

Lentil meatballs

Prep Time: 15 min
Cook Time: 25 min
Servings: 4

INGREDIENTS

- 2.2 oz of grated parmesan cheese
- 11.5 oz of carrots
- 1 clove of garlic
- 3 sprigs fresh parsley
- 2.8 oz Shallot
- 1 oz extra virgin olive oil
- 11.4 oz precooked lentils
- 4.2 oz of bread crumbs
- 2 eggs
- 1/2 teaspoon salt
- 1/2 teaspoon pepper

DIRECTIONS

1. Peel the carrots and cut them into cubes. Wash and dry the parsley. Clean and chop the shallot.
2. Put the carrots, parsley leaves and shallot in a blender and chop.
3. Heat the oil in a saucepan and add the chopped mixture. Leave to gain flavor for a few minutes, add the lentils, breadcrumbs, eggs, salt and pepper. Continue cooking for a few more minutes, stirring well to combine all the ingredients.
4. Preheat the oven to 350°F.
5. Transfer the mixture to a bowl and let it cool, then form 12 meatballs and place them on a baking sheet lined with parchment paper. Sprinkle with a little oil.
6. Bake for 20 minutes.
7. Serve hot or warm.

NUTRITION: Calories: 181.1 cal | Carbs: 17.7 g | Protein: 7.3 g | Fat: 9.5 g | Fiber: 4 |

Italian Grilled Cheese Sandwich

Prep Time: 8 min
Cook Time: 7 min
Servings: 6

INGREDIENTS

- ¼ cup unsalted butter
- ⅛ teaspoon garlic powder
- 12 slices white bread
- 1 teaspoon dried oregano
- 1 (8 ounce) package shredded mozzarella cheese
- 1 (24 ounce) jar vodka marinara sauce

DIRECTIONS

1. Preheat your oven's broiler.
2. On a baking pan, arrange 6 slices of bread. Spread a tiny handful of the mozzarella cheese over each slice. Add the remaining 6 slices of bread on top. Combine the butter and garlic powder in a small bowl, then brush or spread some over the tops of the sandwiches with the back of a tablespoon. Garnish with dried oregano leaves.
3. Broil the baking sheet for 2 to 3 minutes, or until golden brown. Remove skillet from oven, flip sandwiches, brush with butter and sprinkle with oregano on the other side. Return to the broiler and cook for another 2 minutes, or until golden.
4. Cut the sandwiches in half diagonally and serve with vodka.

NUTRITION: Calories 394 Cal | Protein 15g | Carbohydrates 42g | Fat 18.3g | Cholesterol 46.5mg | Sodium 1031.9mg

Tomato Fritters

Prep Time: 20 min
Cook Time: 30 min
Servings: 6

INGREDIENTS

- ¼ cup fresh whole basil leaves
- ½ teaspoon baking powder
- ½ teaspoon kosher salt, plus more for seasoning
- 1 big egg, lightly beaten
- 1 cup all-purpose flour, plus more for dredging
- 6 medium under-ripened tomatoes
- Vegetable oil, for frying

DIRECTIONS

1. Use a deep pot or Dutch oven to heat several inches of oil to 365 degrees. Cut the tomatoes crosswise into ½-inch-thick slices, sprinkle with salt, and drain thoroughly on paper towels, turning once, while making the batter. Cut the basil leaves.
2. In a large container, whisk together the flour, baking powder, and ½ teaspoon salt. Whisk in the egg and ¾ cup water to make a smooth batter. Whisk in the chopped basil barely sufficient to distribute it in the batter.
3. Spread about a cup of flour on a plate. Pat tomatoes dry one more time, then gently dredge them in the flour, on both sides. Immerse in the batter, and fry, in batches, until the batter is puffed and dark golden, approximately 2 minutes per side. Drain on fresh paper towels, and sprinkle lightly with salt. Serve hot.

Italian Cookies

Prep Time: 20 min
Cook Time: 15 min
Servings: 36-48 pcs cookies

- 1/2 cup butter
- 1 1/2 cups granulated sugar
- 5 eggs
- 1/3 cup wine or milk
- 1 1/2 teaspoons anise flavoring
- 4 cups all-purpose flour (or more)
- 1 teaspoon baking powder
- 1/4 teaspoon salt
- 3/4 cup nuts, chopped
- 5 heaping tablespoons confectioners' sugar

1. Preheat oven to 350 degrees F. In a large bowl, cream together butter and sugar. Add eggs (reserving 1 egg white for frosting). Add wine or milk, and anise flavoring. Combine flour, baking powder and salt. Add to creamed mixture; mix well. Stir in nuts.
2. Shape dough into a 1-inch thick roll and place on a cookie sheet. Bake at 350 degrees F. 18 to 20 minutes, until lightly browned. Turn oven off. Mix together reserved egg white with confectioners' sugar. Pour over cookie roll while still hot, then slice at an angle. Return to oven to let dry.

Snacks and Appetizers

Pizza Biscuits

Prep Time 10 min | **Cook Time** 22 min | **Servings** 9

INGREDIENTS

- 1 tablespoon butter, melted
- 1/2 cup tomato sauce
- 1/4 cup chopped onion
- 1 tablespoon canola oil
- 1 garlic clove, minced
- 1/2 teaspoon dried basil
- 1/2 teaspoon dried oregano
- 1 tube (7-1/2 ounces) refrigerated buttermilk biscuits
- 1/3 cup shredded part-skim mozzarella cheese

DIRECTIONS

1. Put butter into a 9-inch square baking pan; put aside. Mix the oregano, basil, garlic, oil, onion and tomato sauce in a bowl. Slice each biscuit into 4 wedges; plunge into the tomato mixture.
2. Put in buttered baking pan; drizzle remaining tomato mixture on top. Dust with mozzarella cheese. Bake for 18-22 minutes at 400° or until golden brown. Serve immediately.

NUTRITION: Calories: 99 Cal | Sodium: 317mg | Fiber: 0 | Total Carbs: 13g | Cholesterol: 6mg | Protein: 3g | Total Fat: 4 g

---

Mussels In Spicy Tomato Sauce

Prep Time 15 min | **Cook Time** 20 min | **Servings** 4-6

INGREDIENTS

- ½ teaspoon dried oregano, preferably Sicilian on the branch
- ½ teaspoon kosher salt
- ½ teaspoon peperoncino flakes
- 10 big fresh basil leaves, shredded
- 3 pounds mussels, scrubbed, debearded, and drained
- 6 tablespoons extra-virgin olive oil
- 8 garlic cloves, sliced
- One 28-ounce can Italian plum tomatoes, preferably San Marzano, crushed by hand or a food mill

DIRECTIONS

1. Heat 5 tablespoons olive oil in a big Dutch oven on moderate to high heat. Put in the sliced garlic, and cook until the garlic sizzles and turns just golden around the edges, approximately 2 minutes. Put in the tomatoes, slosh out the can with ¼ cup water, and put in that to the pot. Season with the oregano, salt, and peperoncino. Bring to its boiling point, and simmer until a little thickened, approximately ten minutes.
2. Once the sauce has thickened, put in the mussels, stir, and adjust the heat so the sauce is simmering. Cover, and simmer until the mussels open, approximately five minutes.
3. Once the mussels have opened (discard any that have not), mix in the basil, and sprinkle with the rest of the tablespoon of olive oil. Move the mussels to a serving container, and pour juices over them. Serve instantly.

Lentil Crostini

Prep Time 15 min | **Cook Time** 45 min | **Servings** 6

INGREDIENTS

- ¼ teaspoon crushed red pepper flakes, or to taste
- 1 cup chopped onion
- 1 cup small lentils, preferably lenticchie di Castelluccio
- 12 slices Italian bread
- 2 cups canned Italian plum tomatoes, preferably San Marzano, crushed by hand
- 2 fresh bay leaves
- 2 medium celery stalks, with leaves, finely chopped (approximately 1 cup)
- 2 plump garlic cloves, sliced
- 2 teaspoons kosher salt
- 6 tablespoons extra-virgin olive oil, plus more for drizzling

DIRECTIONS

1. Wash the lentils, and put them in a big deep cooking pan with the celery, bay leaves, and 3 cups cold water. Bring to its boiling point, cover the pan, and adjust the heat to maintain a gentle, steady simmer. Cook until the lentils are almost tender, approximately twenty minutes (or longer, depending on size).
2. In the meantime, pour 4 tablespoons of the olive oil into a medium frying pan, and set it on moderate heat. Mix in the garlic and onion, and cook for five minutes or more, until the onion is tender and glistening. Drop the red pepper flakes into a hot spot in the pan, and let it toast for one minute; then mix in the crushed tomatoes, season with a teaspoon of the salt, and bring the sauce to a simmer. Let it bubble gently about five minutes, until a little thickened.
3. When the lentils are just a little undercooked, pour the tomato sauce into the deep cooking pan and stir into the lentils. Return the sauce to a simmer, and cook, partially covered, until the lentils are fully cooked and tender, approximately ten minutes. Take the cover, fish out bay leaves, mix in the rest of the teaspoon salt, and let the lentils cook slowly, stirring regularly, until they're very thick and beginning to fall apart, another ten minutes or so. Take the pan from the heat, and mix in the rest of the 2 tablespoons olive oil.
4. For crostini, grill or toast the bread slices, spoon a mound of lentils on each crostino, and sprinkle on slightly of fine olive oil.

Roasted Eggplant Spread with Crackers

Prep Time 25 min | **Cook Time** 50 min | **Servings** 6

INGREDIENTS

- 3 tablespoons (45 ml) olive oil
- 3 cloves garlic, minced
- 2 large bell peppers, sliced
- 1 medium eggplant, cut into 1 inch (2.5 cm) thick pieces
- 1 red onion, sliced
- 1 tablespoon (15 ml) tomato paste
- ½ teaspoon (2.5 ml) salt
- ½ teaspoon (2.5 ml) pepper
- Assorted crackers

DIRECTIONS

1. Preheat your oven to 400° F (205° C)
2. In a large bowl, mix the olive oil, garlic, salt, and pepper.
3. Add the chopped vegetables to the bowl and toss to coat with the oil mixture.
4. Grease a cookie sheet with olive oil or cooking spray and transfer vegetables onto the sheet. Arrange them into an even layer as much as possible for even cooking.
5. Place the vegetables in the oven and roast for 25 minutes. Remove and use a fork to stir the vegetables around, then return the sheet to the oven and roast for an additional 20-25 minutes or until soft and slightly browned.
6. Remove vegetables from the oven and allow to cool for a few minutes.
7. Transfer to a food processor, add tomato paste, and briefly pulse. Your final mixture should be somewhat blended, but still chunky.
8. Transfer to a small bowl and serve with crackers. Spread can be served hot or cold.

Snacks and Appetizers

Lettuce and Bread Quiches

Prep Time 25 min **Cook Time** 22 min **Servings** 10

INGREDIENTS

- ¼ cup bread crumbs
- ½ cup freshly grated Grana Padano
- ½ cup milk
- ¾ teaspoon kosher salt
- 1 bunch scallions, trimmed and chopped (approximately 1 cup)
- 1 tablespoon fresh thyme leaves, chopped
- 1½ cups ½-inch bread cubes
- 3 tablespoons extra-virgin olive oil
- 5 big eggs
- Outer leaves from 1 head romaine lettuce, coarsely chopped (about 3 cups) (save the heart for salad)
- Pinch of freshly grated nutmeg
- Unsalted butter, softened, for lining the muffin tins

DIRECTIONS

1. Preheat your oven to 350 degrees. Brush ten cups of a standard muffin tin with softened butter. Drizzle with the bread crumbs to coat all around, and tap out the surplus.
2. To a big frying pan on moderate to high heat, put in the olive oil. When the oil is hot, put in the scallions and thyme. Season with ½ teaspoon salt. Cook and stir until scallions are wilted, approximately 4 minutes. Put in the lettuce, cover, and cook until wilted, approximately 3 minutes. Uncover, increase heat to high, and cook away any surplus liquid in the pan, approximately one minute. Remove from heat when the lettuce still has a little bite to it. Scrape into a container, and let cool.
3. In a large container, whisk together the eggs, milk, nutmeg, ¼ cup grated cheese, and rest of the ¼ teaspoon salt. Mix in the bread cubes and the cooled lettuce mixture, and let soak five minutes.
4. Spoon solids into the lined muffin cups to distribute uniformly, then pour in the egg mixture. Drizzle the tops with the grated cheese. Bake until golden on top and set throughout, approximately twenty minutes. Cool on a rack for five to ten minutes, then loosen the sides using a paring knife before you serve. These are good warm or at room temperature.
5. Use the crusts from the bread you use for cubes to make the bread crumbs to line the muffin tin. If they are too tender, dry them out in a 350-degree oven for five to ten minutes.

Swordfish-Stuffed Peppers

Prep Time 25 min **Cook Time** 50 min **Servings** 12

- ¼ cup chopped fresh Italian parsley
- ½ cup dry white wine
- 1 teaspoon chopped fresh thyme
- 1 teaspoon kosher salt
- 1 teaspoon kosher salt
- 1¼ pounds skinless swordfish steaks, coarsely chopped
- 1½ cups frozen peas
- 2 bunches scallions, trimmed and coarsely chopped (about 2 cups)
- 4 garlic cloves, finely chopped
- 6 cups crustless day-old bread cubes
- 6 small red, yellow, or orange bell peppers
- 6 tablespoons extra-virgin olive oil

DIRECTIONS

1. Preheat your oven to 400 degrees. Cut each pepper into thirds along the length, along the natural folds. Take the seeds to make 18 pepper "boats." On a rimmed baking sheet, toss the peppers with 2 tablespoons of the olive oil, and season with ½ teaspoon of the salt.
2. Put the bread cubes in a large container, submerge them in water, and allow them to soak while making the stuffing.
3. To a big frying pan on moderate to high heat, put in the rest of the olive oil. When the oil is hot, put in the swordfish, and season with the rest of the ½ teaspoon salt. Stir to coat the swordfish in the oil, then put in the garlic. Once everything is sizzling, mix in the peas and thyme. Put in the wine, and simmer until it has evaporated, approximately five minutes.
4. Put in the scallions, and cook until they are wilted, approximately 3 minutes. Mix in the parsley. Scrape the mixture into a large container. Squeeze all of the water out of the soaked bread, and crumble the bread into the swordfish mixture. Mix thoroughly, and stuff the filling into the pepper boats. Cover with foil, and bake until set, approximately twenty minutes. Uncover, and bake until the top of the filling is golden brown, approximately twenty minutes more. Serve hot or at room temperature.

Pinwheel Pizza Snacks

Prep Time: 15 min
Cook Time: 15 min
Servings: 16

INGREDIENTS

- 1 tube (8 ounces) refrigerated crescent rolls
- 1/3 cup pizza sauce
- 1/4 cup grated Parmesan cheese
- 1/2 cup chopped seeded tomatoes
- 1/3 cup shredded part-skim mozzarella cheese
- Fresh basil leaves, thinly sliced

DIRECTIONS

1. Unroll crescent dough to one long rectangle. Seal perforations and seams. Within 1-in. of edges, spread with pizza sauce. Sprinkle on parmesan cheese. Roll up, beginning with a short side, like a jellyroll. Seal by pinching seams. Cut to 16 slices.
2. Put pinwheels on a greased baking sheet, cut side down. Put mozzarella cheese and tomatoes on each top. Bake for 11-13 minutes or until cheese melts and golden brown at 375 degrees. Sprinkle basil on top.

NUTRITION: Calories: 67Cal | Sodium: 163mg | Fiber: 0 | Carbohydrate: 7g | Cholesterol: 3mg | Protein: 2g | Fat: 3g

Lobster Salad with Fresh Potatoes

Prep Time: 15 min
Cook Time: 10 min
Servings: 6

INGREDIENTS

- ¼ teaspoon peperoncino, or to taste
- ¾ cup extra-virgin olive oil
- 1 teaspoon kosher salt, plus 6 tablespoons for the lobster pot
- 2 big hard-boiled eggs, chopped
- 2 live lobsters, 1¼ pounds each
- 2 tablespoons chopped fresh Italian parsley
- 3 tender celery stalks with a nice amount of leaves
- 4 ripe tomatoes (approximately 1½ pounds), or 1 pound sweet, ripe cherry tomatoes
- Juice of 2 big lemons, freshly squeezed

DIRECTIONS

1. Fill a big stockpot with 6 quarts water, put in 6 tablespoons salt, and bring to a rolling boil. When the water is at a rolling boil, drop in the lobsters and cook them, uncovered, for exactly ten minutes after the water returns to a boil (and then keep it boiling). At the end of ten minutes (or a couple of minutes longer if the lobsters are larger than 1¼ pounds), lift the lobsters from the pot, wash with cold water, drain, and allow them to cool.
2. Core and chop the tomatoes into wedges, approximately 1 inch thick (if you have cherry tomatoes, cut them in half). Cut the celery stalks crosswise into ½-inch pieces, and roughly cut the leaves. Toss the tomatoes and celery together in a big bowl with ½ teaspoon of the salt.
3. When the lobsters are sufficiently cool to handle, twist and pull off the claws and knuckle segments where the knuckles attach to the front of the body. Place the lobsters flat on a cutting board, and cut them in half along the length using a heavy chef's knife. Take the digestive sac, found right behind the eyes, and pull out the vein running along the back of the body and the tail. Cut off the meaty tail piece from the carcass of the four split halves. Take the shell from the upper half of the lobsters, remove the feathered attachments and any surplus skin, and chop the lobster body with small legs attached into three pieces, putting the pieces in a big mixing bowl as you work. It is a good idea to leave the tomalley and roe in the body pieces, as a special treat while eating the salad. Or you can remove them and discard, if not to your preference.
4. Separate the knuckles from the claws, and crack open the shells of both knuckles and hard claw pincers using the thick edge of the knife blade, or kitchen shears; pull the meat out. Get the meat out of the knuckles too. Chop the tail sections, shell on, crosswise into three pieces each.
5. For the dressing, whisk together the lemon juice, chopped eggs, peperoncino, and rest of the ½ teaspoon salt. Pour in the olive oil in a slow stream, whisking continuously to blend it into a smooth dressing.
6. To serve: Put in the tomatoes and celery to the bowl of lobster pieces. Pour in the dressing, and tumble everything together until uniformly coated. Scatter the parsley on top. Position the salad on a big platter, or compose individual servings on salad plates.

Snacks and Appetizers

Panzanella

Prep Time: 20 min
Cook Time: 15 min
Servings: 12

INGREDIENTS

For the salad:
- 2 teaspoons (10 ml) kosher salt
- 2 large, ripe tomatoes, sliced into 1-inch (2 ½ cm) pieces
- 1 small French bread, sliced into 1-inch (2 ½ cm) cubes
- 3 tablespoons (45 ml) extra virgin olive oil
- 1 cucumber, peeled, seeded, cut in half, sliced ½-inch (1 ¼ cm) pieces
- 1 green bell pepper, seeded, sliced into 1-inch (2 ½ cm) pieces
- 1 yellow bell pepper, seeded, sliced into 1-inch (2 ½ cm) pieces
- 1 small red onion, thinly sliced
- ½ bunch basil leaves, chopped

For the dressing:
- 2 cloves garlic, minced
- 3 tablespoons (45 ml) red wine vinegar
- ½ cup (120 ml) extra virgin olive oil
- ½ teaspoon (2.5 ml) kosher salt
- ¼ teaspoon (1.25 ml) freshly ground black pepper

DIRECTIONS

1. Program your oven to 350° F (175° C)
2. Place the tomatoes into a colander set over a bowl, sprinkle two teaspoons of kosher salt over them and allow the tomatoes to sit for 15 minutes.
3. Place the cubed French bread onto a cookie sheet, drizzle the olive oil on top and toss to combine. Bake the bread for 15 minutes until crispy.
4. To make the vinaigrette, remove the tomatoes from the bowl and set them aside. Add the garlic, red wine vinegar, olive oil salt, and pepper and whisk to combine.
5. Place the tomatoes, cucumber, green and yellow bell peppers, red onion, basil, and bread cubes into a large bowl.
6. Add the vinaigrette and toss to combine.
7. Serve and enjoy!

Garlic Risotto Stuffed Mushrooms

Prep Time: 10 min
Cook Time: 50 min
Servings: 32

- 2 tablespoons (30 ml) olive oil
- 1 shallot, minced
- 3 cloves garlic, minced
- ¾ cup (175 ml) arborio rice
- 1 teaspoon (5 ml) salt
- ½ teaspoon (2.5 ml) white pepper
- 2 tablespoons (30 ml) Pinot Grigio or another dry white wine
- 2 cups (470 ml) low-sodium vegetable broth
- 1 tablespoon (15 ml) nutritional yeast
- 32 cremini mushrooms, washed, drained, stems removed
- 1 tablespoon (15 ml) freshly minced parsley

DIRECTIONS

1. Place the oil into a heavy bottom skillet over medium-high heat. Add the shallot and sauté for 2 minutes until it is translucent.
2. Add the garlic and arborio rice and sauté it for another 2-3 minutes until it is slightly translucent.
3. Add the Pinot Grigio and cook it for 2 minutes until the wine evaporates. Add the vegetable broth, salt, and white pepper, stir to combine, and allow the risotto to come to a boil.
4. Decrease the flame to medium-low, place the lid on the skillet, and cook for 20 minutes cook until most of the vegetable broth is absorbed.
5. Remove the garlic risotto from the heat and stir in the nutritional yeast.
6. Arrange the cremini mushrooms onto a cooking sheet cap side up.
7. Add one heaping tablespoon (>15ml) of the garlic risotto to each cremini mushroom and bake it for 20 minutes until the mushrooms are tender.
8. Sprinkle the parsley over the garlic risotto stuffed mushrooms.
9. Serve and enjoy!

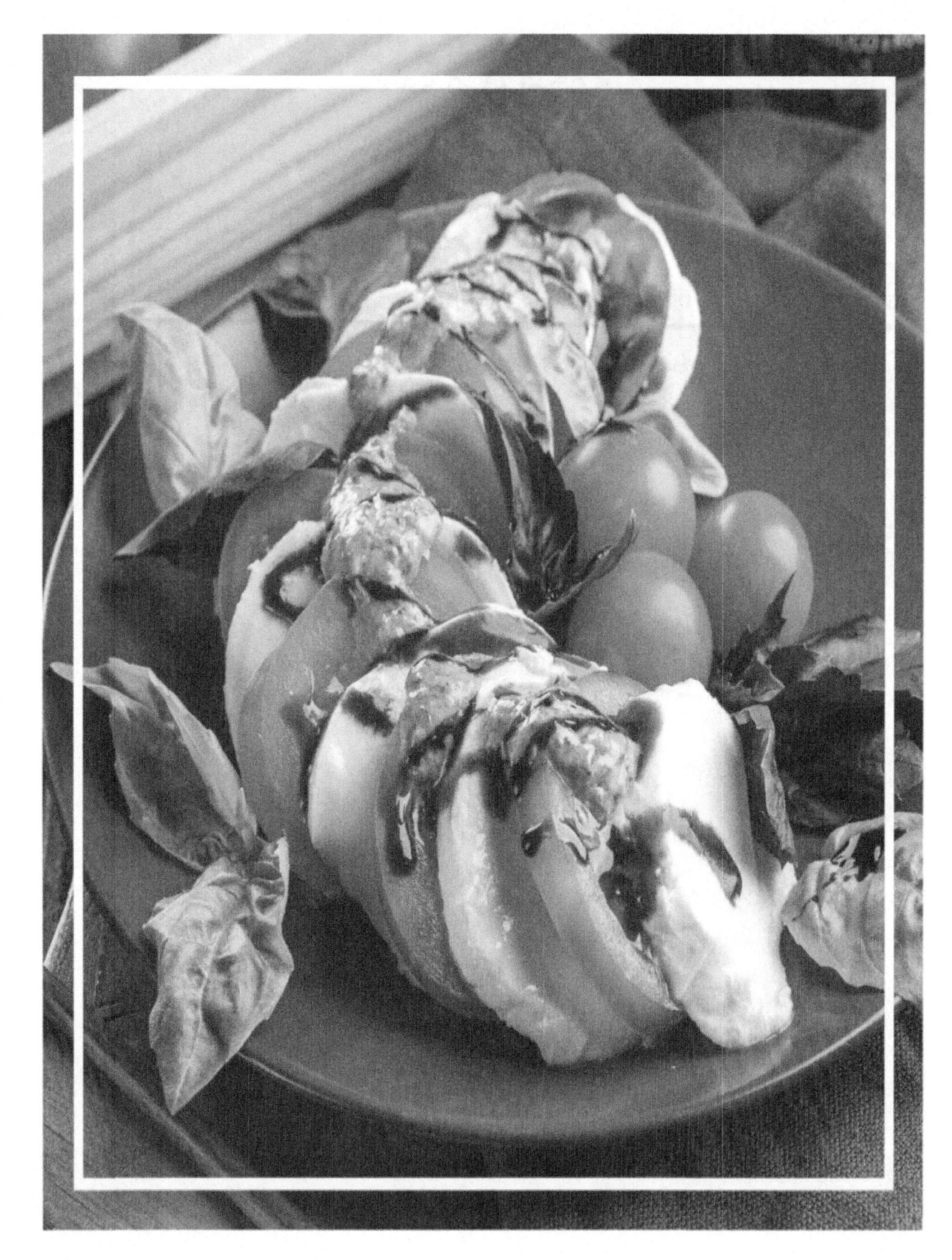

Salads

Basil Garden Salad

Prep Time: 15 min | **Cook Time:** 0 min | **Servings:** 6

INGREDIENTS
- 2 cups torn leaf lettuce
- 1 cup torn Bibb lettuce
- 3 green onions with tops, sliced
- 1 medium tomato, peeled and diced
- 6 fresh mushrooms, sliced
- 9 fresh basil leaves, thinly sliced
- 2 tablespoons red wine vinegar
- 3 tablespoons olive oil
- 1/4 teaspoon pepper
- 1/2 teaspoon salt, optional
- 1/2 teaspoon sugar, optional

DIRECTIONS
1. Mix basil, mushrooms, tomato, onions, and lettuce in a big salad bowl. Blend sugar (optional), salt, pepper, oil, and vinegar in a jar with a tight lid. Cover then shake well. Pour on salad while tossing to coat. Serve quickly.

NUTRITION: Calories: 78 Cal | Total Carbohydrate: 3g | Cholesterol: 0 | Protein: 1g | Fat: 7g | Sodium: 6mg

---

Cherry Tomato Corn Salad

Prep Time: 15 min | **Cook Time:** 0 min | **Servings:** 4

INGREDIENTS
- 1/4 cup minced fresh basil
- 3 tablespoons olive oil
- 2 teaspoons lime juice
- 1 teaspoon sugar
- 1/2 teaspoon salt
- 1/4 teaspoon pepper
- 2 cups frozen corn, thawed
- 2 cups cherry tomatoes, halved
- 1 cup chopped seeded peeled cucumber

DIRECTIONS
1. Mix pepper, salt, sugar, lime juice, oil and basil together in a jar that has a tight-fitting lid. Thoroughly shake.
2. Mix tomatoes, cucumber and corn together in a big bowl. Drizzle the dressing over; mix to coat. Chill until enjoying.

NUTRITION: Calories: 125 | Sodium: 302mg | Fiber: 2g | Carbohydrate: 15g | Protein: 2g | Fat: 7g

Cherry Tomato Salad

Prep Time: 15 min | **Cook Time**: 5 min | **Servings**: 6

INGREDIENTS

- 40 cherry tomatoes, halved
- 1 cup pitted and sliced green olives
- 1 (6 ounce) can black olives, drained and sliced
- 2 green onions, minced
- 3 ounces pine nuts
- 1/2 cup olive oil
- 2 tablespoons red wine vinegar
- 1 tablespoon white sugar
- 1 teaspoon dried oregano
- salt and pepper to taste

DIRECTIONS

1. Mix spring onion, black olives, green olives and cherry tomatoes together in a big bowl.
2. Toast pine nuts in a dry skillet over medium heat until turning golden brown, flipping often. Mix into the tomato mixture.
3. Combine oregano, sugar, red wine vinegar and olive oil in a small bowl. Use pepper and salt to season to taste. Add onto the salad, and gently mix to coat. Refrigerate for 60 minutes.

NUTRITION: Calories: 341 Cal | Sodium: 940 | Cholesterol: 0 | Protein: 5.1 | Fat: 32.2

Arugula Salad With Shaved Parmesan

Prep Time: 15 min | **Cook Time**: 0 min | **Servings**: 4

INGREDIENTS

- 6 cups fresh arugula
- 1/4 cup golden raisins
- 1/4 cup sliced almonds, toasted
- 3 tablespoons olive oil
- 1 tablespoon lemon juice
- 1/4 teaspoon salt
- 1/4 teaspoon freshly ground pepper
- 1/3 cup shaved or shredded Parmesan cheese

DIRECTIONS

1. Mix together almonds, raisins and arugula in a big bowl. Pour lemon juice and oil over. Sprinkle with pepper and salt then toss to coat well. Split among 4 plates and sprinkle with cheese on top.

NUTRITION: Calories: 181 Cal | Protein: 4g | Total Fat: 15g | Sodium: 242mg | Fiber: 2g | Total Carbs: 10g | Cholesterol: 4mg

Salads

Vegetable Salad

Prep Time: 30 min
Cook Time: 0 min
Servings: 12

INGREDIENTS

- 1 cup cut fresh green beans
- 1 cup fresh sugar snap peas
- 1 cup sliced yellow summer squash
- 1 cup sliced zucchini
- 1/2 cup julienned onion
- 2 small tomatoes, seeded and chopped
- 1 cup coarsely grated carrots
- 2/3 cup reduced-fat Italian salad dressing
- 4 teaspoons minced chives
- 2 teaspoons dried basil

DIRECTIONS

1. Boil 2 in. of water in a saucepan. Put in onion, zucchini, yellow squash, peas and beans. Lower heat; cover up and let it simmer till veggies are tender-crisp or for 2 to 3 minutes. Drain off; wash in cold water and pat dry.
2. Transfer veggies in a bowl; put in the leftover ingredients. Coat by lightly mixing. Keep chilled in refrigerator till serving.

NUTRITION: Calories: 47 Cal | Cholesterol: 0 | Protein: 1g | Total Fat: 2g | Sodium: 132mg | Carbohydrate: 6g

---

Artichoke Red Pepper Tossed Salad

Prep Time: 15 min
Cook Time: 0 min
Servings: 20

INGREDIENTS

- 1 head medium head iceberg lettuce
- 1 bunch romaine, torn
- 1 can (14 ounces) water-packed artichoke hearts, rinsed, drained and chopped
- 2 medium sweet red peppers, julienned
- 1/2 cup thinly sliced red onion
- 1/2 cup olive oil
- 1/2 cup red wine vinegar
- 2 tablespoons Dijon mustard
- 2 teaspoons sugar
- 1 teaspoon seasoned salt
- 1/2 cup shredded Parmesan cheese

DIRECTIONS

1. Combine the initial 5 ingredients in a large bowl. Combine seasoned salt, sugar, mustard, vinegar and oil in a jar, cover with a tight-fitting lid and shake well. Drizzle the salad with dressing and toss till coated. Sprinkle Parmesan cheese over.

Copper Carrot Salad

Prep Time: 10 min
Cook Time: 25 min
Servings: 16

INGREDIENTS

- 5 pounds carrots, cut into 1/4-inch slices
- 2 medium green peppers, chopped
- 1 large onion, chopped
- 2 cans (10-3/4 ounces each) condensed tomato soup, undiluted
- 1-1/2 cups sugar
- 1-1/2 cups vinegar
- 1 cup vegetable oil
- 2 tablespoons Italian seasoning
- 2 teaspoons ground mustard
- 2 teaspoons curry powder
- 2 teaspoons Worcestershire sauce
- 1/2 teaspoon salt
- 1/2 teaspoon pepper

DIRECTIONS

1. Put carrots in a Dutch oven. Pour in 1 inch of water. Boil. Lower the heat; simmer with a cover till the carrots turn tender, 15-20 minutes. Strain; rinse in cold water.
2. Mix carrots, onion and green peppers in a large bowl; set aside. Mix together the remaining ingredients in a large saucepan; cook over medium heat, stirring occasionally, till the sugar dissolves. Allow to cool for 10 minutes. Transfer over the carrot mixture; toss to coat. Refrigerate with a cover for 24 hours. Serve accompanied by a slotted spoon.

NUTRITION: Calories: 278 Cal | Fat: 14g | Sodium: 244mg | Fiber: 5g | Carbohydrate: 38g | Cholesterol: 0 | Protein: 2g

---

Corn Pasta Salad

Prep Time: 20 min
Cook Time: 0 min
Servings: 10

INGREDIENTS

- 2 cups cooked tricolor spiral pasta
- 1 package (16 ounces) frozen corn, thawed
- 1 cup chopped celery
- 1 medium green pepper, chopped
- 1 cup chopped seeded tomatoes
- 1/2 cup diced pimientos
- 1/2 cup chopped red onion
- 1 cup picante sauce
- 2 tablespoons canola oil
- 1 tablespoon lemon juice
- 1 garlic clove, minced
- 1 tablespoon sugar
- 1/2 teaspoon salt

DIRECTIONS

1. Mix the first 7 ingredients in a big bowl. Mix together the salt, sugar, garlic, lemon juice, oil and picante sauce in a jar with a tight-fitting lid, then shake well.
2. Drizzle the dressing over the pasta mixture and toss well to coat. Cover and chill overnight

NUTRITION: Calories: 133 Cal | Cholesterol: 0 | Protein: 3g | Fat: 3g | Sodium: 301mg | Fiber: 3g | Carbs: 24g

Salads

Corn Relish Salad

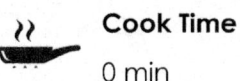

Prep Time 20 min **Cook Time** 0 min **Servings** 10

INGREDIENTS

- 2 cups fresh corn
- 3 medium seeded tomatoes, chopped
- 1 medium green pepper, diced
- 1/2 cup red onion, chopped
- 6-1/2 ounces marinated artichoke hearts, undrained
- 2-1/4 ounces, ripe olives, sliced and drained
- 1/4 cup reduced-fat Italian salad dressing
- 1 tsp. dried basil
- Half teaspoon garlic powder
- Half teaspoon dried oregano
- 1/4 teaspoon lemon-pepper seasoning

DIRECTIONS

1. Mix the first 6 ingredients in a big bowl. Mix lemon-pepper, artichoke, oregano, salad dressing, garlic powder, and basil in a separate bowl; gently toss into the corn mixture. Cover then chill for at least 6 hrs then serve.

NUTRITION: Calories: 68 Cal | Total Carbs: 13g | Cholesterol: 1mg | Protein: 2g | Total Fat: 2g | Sodium: 193mg | Fiber: 2g

---

Sicilian Salad

Prep Time 30 min **Cook Time** 30 min **Servings** 10

INGREDIENTS

- 3 bunches arugula (3/4 lb), coarse stems discarded and leaves torn into pieces
- 1/2 lb Bibb lettuce (2 small heads), leaves torn if large
- 1 celery heart (1/2 lb), thinly sliced on a sharp diagonal
- 1 small red onion, halved lengthwise and very thinly sliced crosswise
- 1/2 lb cherry tomatoes, halved
- 1/2 lb brine-cured black olives (1 cup), drained
- 2 tablespoons drained bottled capers, rinsed
- 1/3 cup extra-virgin olive oil
- 1 teaspoon coarse sea salt (preferably Sicilian)
- 2 tablespoons red-wine vinegar

DIRECTIONS

1. To prepare: In a big bowl, mix together the capers, olives, tomatoes, onion, celery, lettuce and arugula. Drizzle the greens with oil and sprinkle sea salt on top, then give it a toss. Drizzle with vinegar and toss well again.
2. Cooks' notes: If the sea salt you're using is pebblelike and very granular, crush it with the bottom of a heavy skillet or the flat side of a big heavy knife.
3. (You can wash and tear the greens 1 day in advance and chilled in closed plastic bags lined with wet paper towels.)

NUTRITION: Calories: 101 | Total Fat: 9 g | Saturated Fat: 1 g | Sodium: 313 mg | Fiber: 2 g | Total Carbohydrate: 5 g

Sweet Sour Pasta Salad

Prep Time 30 min   **Cook Time** 0 min   **Servings** 16

INGREDIENTS

- 1 package (16 ounces) tricolor spiral pasta
- 1 medium red onion, chopped
- 1 medium tomato, chopped
- 1 medium cucumber, peeled, seeded and chopped
- 1 medium green pepper, chopped
- 2 tablespoons minced fresh parsley

Dressing:
- 1-1/2 cups sugar
- 1/2 cup white vinegar
- 1 tablespoon ground mustard
- 1 teaspoon salt, optional
- 1 teaspoon garlic powder

DIRECTIONS

1. Follow the package directions to cook the pasta, then drain and rinse under cold water. Put in a big serving bowl. Stir in parsley, green pepper, cucumber, tomato and onion, then set aside.
2. Mix the dressing ingredients in a small saucepan, then cook on moderately low heat, until the sugar has dissolved or for 10 minutes. Drizzle over salad and toss to coat well. Chill, covered, for 2 hours, then serve with a slotted spoon.

NUTRITION: Calories: 137 Cal | Sodium: 5mg | Fiber: 0 g | Carbs: 21g | Protein: 11g | Fat: 1g

---

Warm Shrimp Salad with Kamut

Prep Time 30 min   **Cook Time** 10 min   **Servings** 4

INGREDIENTS

- 3 eco-friendly apples, 2 diced and also 1 very finely cut For garnish.
- 7 oz. (200 g) radicchio, thinly sliced.
- 10 1/2 oz. (300 g) poultry breast.
- 3 1/2 oz. (100 g) focaccia, cut into cubes.
- 1/4 cup (20 g) sliced almonds.
- 1/3 cup plus 1 1/2 tbsp. (100 ml) extra-virgin olive oil.
- 1 tablespoon. Plus 1 tsp. (20 ml).
- Vinegar.
- Salt and pepper.

DIRECTIONS

1. Bring a small Saucepan of salty water to a boil. Include peas and cook them until simply tender. Drain and also rinse peas under cold water.
2. Warmth 1 tbsp. plus 2 tsp. of oil in a frying pan over medium warm. Add onion and also chef, mixing, till tender. Add zucchini and also carrots and season with Salt and pepper. Cook till lightly browned however not softened. Include blanched peas. Eliminate from heat.
3. boil spelt in salted water, stress it and place it in a bowl. Include cooked vegetables, tomato, parsley, as well as hand-torn basil. Drizzle with olive oil and also Salt to taste. Sauté shrimp in a little oil as well as serve them with spelt salad.

Salads

Zucchini Orzo Salad

Prep Time: 20 min
Cook Time: 15 min
Servings: 4

INGREDIENTS

- 2 zucchinis, quartered lengthwise and sliced
- 1 cup of orzo
- 4 tsp. of olive oil
- 1 garlic clove, chopped
- 1 tbsp. of white wine
- ½ cup of fresh basil leaves
- Salt and ground pepper

DIRECTIONS

1. Cook the orzo until al dente in salted boiling water, then drain. Spread them on a baking sheet and cool. Cook the zucchini in 1 tablespoon of hot oil until tender and season with salt and pepper. Mix the vinegar, orzo, basil, 1 tablespoon of oil, orzo in a bowl, and cover using a wrap. Refrigerate for an hour before serving.

Antipasto Pasta Salad

Prep Time: 20 min
Cook Time: 15 min
Servings: 12

INGREDIENTS

- 1 pound seashell pasta
- 1 (tree fourth oz.) package dry Italian-style salad dressing mix
- 1/4 pound Genoa salami, chopped
- 3/4 cup extra virgin olive oil
- 1/4 pound pepperoni sausage, chopped
- 1/4 cup balsamic vinegar
- 1/2 pound Asiago cheese, diced
- 6 tsp. dried oregano
- 1 (6oz) can black olives, drained and chopped
- 1 tablespoon dried parsley
- 1 red bell pepper, diced
- 1 tbsp. grated Parmesan cheese
- 1 green bell pepper, chopped
- salt and ground black pepper to taste
- 3 medium tomatoes, chopped
- 1 (3/4 oz.) package dry Italian-style salad dressing mix

DIRECTIONS

1. Cook the pasta till al dente in a big pot of salted boiling water. Drain and rinse under cold water to cool.
2. Toss together the spaghetti, salami, pepperoni, Asiago cheese, black olives, red bell pepper, green bell pepper, and tomatoes in a large mixing basin. Mix in the dressing mix envelope. Refrigerate for at least one hour after covering.
3. Whisk together the olive oil, balsamic vinegar, oregano, parsley, Parmesan cheese, salt, and pepper to make the dressing. Pour the dressing over the salad just before serving and toss well.

NUTRITION: Calories: 451 | Carbos: 33.2g | Fat: 29.1g | Protein: 15g | Cholesterol: 37mg

Fusilli Pasta Salad with Vegetable and Squid

Prep Time 15 min **Cook Time** 10 min **Servings** 4

INGREDIENTS

- 14 oz. (400 g) fusilli.
- 3 1/2 oz. (100 g) carrots or concerning 2 tiny, peeled 12 1/2 oz. (360 g) zucchini, or about 3 tiny.
- 10 1/2 oz. (300 g) artichokes.
- 10 1/2 oz. (300 g) squid Leafy herbs, as needed.
- 1/4 mug (60 ml) extra-virgin olive oil.
- Juice of 1 lemon Salt as well as white pepper 3 1/2 oz. (100 g)

DIRECTIONS

1. Swiss chard, sliced remove difficult outer leaves from artichokes. Cut each artichokes in half lengthwise as well as scoop out fuzzy choke with a melon sphere cutter. In a bowl, combine water and also a few of lemon juice. Reduce artichokes into narrow strips and also let take in lemon juice mix to stop them from browning reduce carrots and zucchini right into thin, narrow strips tidy squid by getting rid of skin from body and reducing arms from body. Flip back arms as well as squeeze out and throw out beak located in center of tentacles. Eliminate eyes, entrails, and transoms and dad inner cartilage. Then cut body right into really slim strips.
2. Bring a pot of well-salted water to a boil. Add pasta, and also 5 minutes before it is cooked, add veggies to water. Mix and also cook For 3 minutes, after that add squid for last 2 minutes drainpipe, include a little oil, and transfer every little thing to a tray and also to cool. When awesome, outfit with rest of oil and lemon juice, and also period with Salt and white pepper. Serve on a bed of fresh aromatic natural herbs as well as Swiss chard.

Seashell Salad

Prep Time 20 min **Cook Time** 0 min **Servings** 6

INGREDIENTS

- 3 cups uncooked medium shell, spiral and/or wagon wheel pasta
- 1/3 cup vinegar
- 1/4 cup olive oil
- 1 teaspoon garlic salt
- 1 teaspoon sugar
- 1 teaspoon Italian seasoning
- 1/4 teaspoon pepper
- 1 medium sweet red pepper
- 1 medium sweet yellow pepper
- 2 tablespoons chopped green onions

DIRECTIONS

1. Follow the package directions to cook the pasta until tender, then drain and rinse under cold water. Transfer into a big bowl, then set aside. Mix together seasonings, oil and vinegar in a jar with a tight-fitting lid and shake well. Put the peppers, dressing and onions into the pasta, then toss to coat well. Cover and chill until serving

NUTRITION: Calories: 222 Cal | Cholesterol: 0 | Protein: 6g | Total Fat: 8g | Sodium: 230mg | Carbs: 33g

Salads

Caesar Salad

Prep Time: 15 min
Cook Time: 1 hour and 10 min
Servings: 8

INGREDIENTS

- 1/4 cup grated Parmesan cheese
- 1/4 cup mayonnaise
- 2 tablespoons milk
- 1 tablespoon lemon juice
- 1 tablespoon Dijon-mayonnaise blend
- 1 garlic clove, minced
- Dash cayenne pepper
- 1 bunch romaine, torn
- Salad croutons and additional grated Parmesan cheese, optional

DIRECTIONS

1. Combine the initial 7 ingredients together by whisking them in a small bowl. In a big bowl, set the romaine down. Pour the dressing over it in a drizzling motion, tossing until coated. If desired, put extra cheese and salad croutons on the top before serving.

NUTRITION: Calories: 73 Cal | Total Carbs: 2g | Protein: 2g protein | Total Fat: 6g | Sodium: 126mg | Fiber: 1g

---

Deli Pasta Salad With Veggies

Prep Time: 25 min
Cook Time: 0 min
Servings: 20

INGREDIENTS

- 1 package (1 pound) ziti, penne, bow tie or tricolor spiral pasta
- 2 large cucumbers, peeled, seeded and chopped
- 2 large red onions, sliced into thin strips
- 2 large green peppers, chopped
- 2 large tomatoes, chopped
- 1 bottle (16 ounces) Italian salad dressing
- 1 container (2.6 ounces) Salad Supreme Seasoning

DIRECTIONS

1. Follow the package directions to cook the pasta, then drain and rinse under cold water.
2. Mix together the tomatoes, green peppers, onions, cucumbers and pasta in a big bowl. Whisk the seasoning and salad dressing in a small bowl, then drizzle over pasta mixture and toss to coat well. Cover and chill for a minimum of 1 hour. Gently toss right before serving.

NUTRITION: Calories: 152 | Sodium: 312mg | Fiber: 2g fiber) | Total Carbs: 19g | Protein: 3g protein | Fat: 7g

Desserts and Fruits

Watermelon Granita

Prep Time: 15 min
Freezing Time: 2 h 30 min
Cook Time: 0
Servings: 8

INGREDIENTS
- 1 lb. (0.5 kg) (1.6 cups/385 ml) watermelon, rind removed, cut into small pieces
- 2 tablespoons (30 ml) granulated sugar
- 2 tablespoons (30 ml) maple syrup
- 2 tablespoons (30 ml) lemon juice

DIRECTIONS
1. Arrange the watermelon pieces on a parchment-lined cookie sheet and freeze them until frozen solid.
2. Place the frozen watermelon cubes, sugar, maple syrup, and lemon juice into a blender and blend it until smooth.
3. Pour the watermelon granita into a shallow baking dish and freeze it for 2 1/2 hours, raking a fork through the granita every 30 minutes until it is slushy and crunchy.
4. Serve and enjoy!

White Chocolate Macadamia Biscotti

Prep Time: 15 min
Cook Time: 25 min
Servings: 3-4 dozen

INGREDIENTS
- 3/4 cup granulated sugar
- 1/2 cup butter
- 2 eggs
- 2 tablespoons Amaretto liqueur
- 1 teaspoon vanilla extract
- 2 cups + 2 tablespoons all-purpose flour, divided
- 1 1/2 teaspoons baking powder
- 1/4 teaspoon salt
- 2/3 cup macadamia nuts, chopped
- 2/3 cup white chocolate chips

DIRECTIONS
1. Preheat oven to 325 degrees F. In a large mixing bowl, cream sugar and butter until light and fluffy. Beat in eggs, Amaretto liqueur and vanilla. In a separate bowl, combine 2 cups flour, baking powder and salt. Add to creamed mixture, blending well. Fold in nuts and chocolate chips.
2. Divide dough in half. On a greased and floured baking sheet, pat out dough into 2 logs about 1/2-inch high, 1 1/2-inch wide and 14-inch long, spacing them at least 2 inches apart. Bake at 325 degrees F. for 25 minutes, or until lightly browned. Remove from oven; transfer from baking sheet to a wire rack. Cool for 5 minutes.
3. Place biscotti on a cutting board. Use a serrated knife to slice 1/2-inch thick slices diagonally at a 45-degree angle. Return the slices upright to the baking sheet. Bake for an additional 8 minutes to dry slightly. Let cool on a rack

Sicilian Chocolate Cake

Prep Time 15 min | **Freezing Time:** 2 hours | **Cook Time** 0 | **Servings** 8

INGREDIENTS

Cake:
- 1 9x3-inch pound cake
- 1 lb. ricotta cheese
- 2 tablespoons heavy cream
- 1/4 cup granulated sugar
- 3 tablespoons orange-flavored liqueur
- 3 tablespoons candied fruit, coarsely chopped
- 2 oz. semi-sweet chocolate pieces

Frosting:
- 12 oz. semi-sweet chocolate chips
- 3/4 cup strong black coffee
- 1/2 lb. unsalted butter, cut into 1/2-inch pieces, thoroughly chilled

DIRECTIONS

Cake:
1. 1 9x3-inch pound cake
2. 1 lb. ricotta cheese
3. 2 tablespoons heavy cream
4. 1/4 cup granulated sugar
5. 3 tablespoons orange-flavored liqueur
6. 3 tablespoons candied fruit, coarsely chopped
7. 2 oz. semi-sweet chocolate pieces

Frosting:

8. 12 oz. semi-sweet chocolate chips
9. 3/4 cup strong black coffee
10. 1/2 lb. unsalted butter, cut into 1/2-inch pieces, thoroughly chilled

Mediterranean fennel cakes

Prep Time 10 min | **Cook Time** 30 min | **Servings** 4

INGREDIENTS

- Fennels 21.7 oz
- Cherry tomatoes 7 oz
- Edamer cheese 2.8 oz
- Salted capers 0.5 oz
- Black olives pitted 8
- Breadcrumbs 0.7 oz

DIRECTIONS

1. To make the Mediterranean style fennel cakes, thinly slice the fennels using a mandoline.
2. Wash the cherry tomatoes and cut them into thin slices.
3. Cut the cheese into cubes.
4. Take some 4 inch diameter aluminum ramekins with a 1.2 inch high rim. Melt the butter and butter the bottom and rim with the help of a kitchen brush. Dust the entire inside surface with breadcrumbs.
5. Fill your ramekins: place a layer of fennels on the bottom, then one of cherry tomatoes and season with capers (previously desalinated), a few cheese cubes and olives cut into rounds. Now cover with another layer of fennels.
6. Spread some breadcrumbs and a piece of butter on top.
7. Place your ramekins on a baking sheet and bake in a static oven preheated to 356°F for 30 minutes, including the last 5 minutes with the grill function. When cooked, the Mediterranean style fennel cakes will be nicely au gratin, serve them warm!

NUTRITION Calories: 180 cal. | Carbs: 6.4 g. | Protein: 7.6 g. | Fat: 13.8 g. | Fiber: 2.6 g.

Savory Biscuits

Prep Time: 15 min
Cook Time: 30 min
Servings: 8

- 2 tubes (12 ounces each) refrigerated buttermilk biscuits
- 1/2 cup shredded Monterey Jack cheese
- 1/2 cup shredded cheddar cheese
- 3 tablespoons butter, melted
- 3/4 teaspoon dried basil
- 1/4 teaspoon dried oregano
- 1/8 teaspoon dill weed
- 1/8 teaspoon garlic powder

1. Divide each tube of biscuits into 10 biscuits; put a single layer in a greased 11x7-in. baking pan. Dust with cheeses. Drizzle using butter; sprinkle with seasonings. Bake at 350 degrees until golden brown, or for 25-30 minutes. Serve warm.

NUTRITION: Calories: 77 | Sodium: 195mg | Fiber: 0 | Carbohydrate: 8g | Protein: 3g | Fat: 4g

---

Apple Strudel

Prep Time: 1 hour
Cook Time: 1 hour and 5 min
Servings: 4

For dough
- 2 mugs (250 g) all-purpose flour.
- 2/3 cup (150 ml) water.
- 4 tablespoon. (20 ml) extra-virgin olive oil.
- Squeeze salt.

For filling
- 1 3/4 pounds. (800 g) apples.
- 3 1/2 oz. (100 g) raisins.
- 3 1/2 oz. (100 g) ache nuts, or regarding 2/3 cup.
- 1/2 stick (57 g) unsalted butter.
- 2-3 1/2 oz. (57-100 g) breadcrumbs, or 1/2 -1 cup.
- cinnamon, as needed.

For designing
- 1 large egg
- confectioners' sugar, as required.

1. Mix flour with water, oil and Salt on a job surface and knead up until dough is smooth as well as homogeneous. create it into a sphere, cover with cling wrap, and let rest For a minimum of 30 minutes
2. At same time, prepare loading For strudel. Peel and also cut apples. saturate raisins in a bowl of warm water For 15 minutes; then drain raisins and press to remove excess water.
3. Melt butter in a big frying pan. Include apple slices, raisins, yearn nuts, and also a pinch cinnamon. stir in adequate breadcrumbs to reach your wanted filling up uniformity. Heat stove to 350 ° F (180 ° C) and also line a cooking sheet with parchment. with rear of your hands, stretch dough right into a slim sheet on a gently floured work surface area. spoon filling up along lengthy side of pastry, leaving a 2 inches (couple of cm) border as well as roll it up, making sure it is well secured by pushing down along edges with your fingers as well as curling up both ends.
4. in a little bowl, lightly defeat egg with a fork. Brush strudel with egg. established it on ready flat pan and cook For about 20 minutes A few minutes before it is done, dust with powdered sugar and also coating cooking. serve with whipped lotion, if you such as.

Desserts and Fruits

Almond Italian Cookies

Prep Time: 10 min **Cook Time:** 25 min **Servings:** 8

INGREDIENTS
- 1 cup almond flakes
- 5 eggs
- 4 tablespoon strawberry jam
- 1 teaspoon vanilla extract
- ¼ teaspoon almond extract
- 2 cup almond flour
- ½ cup sugar
- ¼ teaspoon salt

DIRECTIONS
1. Beat 4 eggs in the mixer bowl and whisk them.
2. Add almond flour and strawberry jam.
3. After this, add salt and vanilla extract.
4. Knead the non-sticky dough.
5. Whisk the egg in the bowl.
6. Make the log from the almond flour dough and cut it into the small balls.
7. Then deep the almond flour balls in the whisked egg.
8. After this, coat the almond flour balls in the almond flakes.
9. Preheat the oven to 365 F.
10. Put the cookies on the tray and cook them for 25 minutes.
11. Then chill the cookies very well.
12. Serve the dish immediately.

NUTRITION: Calories 112 Cal | Fat 6.3g | Fiber 0 | Carbohydrates 7.5g | **Protein** 6g

---

Fresh Orange Gelato

Prep Time: 15 min **Cook Time:** 0 min **Servings:** 4

INGREDIENTS
- 2 eggs + 2 egg yolks
- 3/4 cup + 2 tablespoons granulated sugar
- 2 cups orange juice, freshly squeezed
- 3 cups heavy whipping cream
- Juice of 2 lemons
- 1/2 teaspoon vanilla extract

DIRECTIONS
1. Use an electric mixer to beat eggs, egg yolks and sugar until pale and creamy. Add orange juice, whipping cream, lemon juice and vanilla. Blend together. Transfer mixture to an ice cream maker and freeze. If you're not using an ice cream freezer, freeze mixture in a shallow pan until almost solid, then blend in a food processor. Place mixture in freezer to finish freezing.

Panucci Fudge

Prep Time: 15 min **Cook Time:** 35 min **Servings:** 5

INGREDIENTS
- 1 cup granulated sugar
- 3/4 cup milk
- 2 cups brown sugar, packed
- 1/8 tsp. cream of tartar
- 2 tbsp. light corn syrup
- 1/8 tsp. salt
- 1/4 cup butter, divided
- 1 tsp. vanilla extract

DIRECTIONS
1. Mix the granulated sugar, milk, brown sugar, cream of tartar, corn syrup, and salt
2. Over medium heat, stirring constantly. Continue cooking without stirring until candy reaches the softball stage (about 236 degrees F.).
3. Remove pan and, without stirring, add butter and vanilla.
4. Cool for about 30 minutes before beating.
5. Then beat by hand until it begins to thicken and gloss disappears.
6. Pour into an 8 x 8-inch buttered pan.

Tiramisu Layer Cake

Prep Time: 5 min
Cook Time: 20 min
Servings: 12

- 1 (18.25 ounce) package moist white cake mix
- 1 (8 ounce) container mascarpone cheese
- 1 teaspoon instant coffee powder
- 1/2 cup confectioners' sugar
- 1/4 cup coffee
- 2 tablespoons coffee flavored liqueur
- 1 tablespoon coffee flavored liqueur
- 1/4 cup confectioners' sugar
- 2 cups heavy cream
- 2 tablespoons coffee flavored liqueur
- 2 tablespoons unsweetened cocoa powder
- 1 (1 ounce) square semisweet chocolate

1. Preheat the oven to 350 degrees Fahrenheit (175 degrees C). 3 (9-inch) pans, greased and floured
2. Follow the package directions for making the cake mix. Two-thirds of the batter should be divided between two pans. Pour the remaining batter into the remaining pan, stirring in the instant coffee.
3. Bake for 20 to 25 minutes in a preheated oven or until a toothpick inserted in the center of the cake comes out clean. Allow cooling for 10 minutes in the pan before turning out onto a wire rack to cool completely. Combine brewed coffee and 1 tablespoon coffee liqueur in a measuring cup and put aside.
4. To create the frosting, whisk the cream, 1/4 cup confectioners' sugar, and 2 tablespoons coffee liqueur until stiff in a medium bowl with an electric mixer set on medium-high speed. 1/2 cup of the cream mixture should be folded into the filling mixture.
5. Place a layer of coffee-flavored cake on top and poke holes in it. Over the second layer, pour another third of the coffee mixture and spread the remaining filling. Place the remaining cake layer on top and poke holes in it. Pour the rest of the coffee mixture on top. Apply frosting to the sides and top of the cake. Using a sieve, lightly dust the top of the cake with cocoa powder. Serve with chocolate curls as a garnish. Before serving, chill for at least 30 minutes.
6. Use a vegetable peeler to run along the edge of the chocolate bar to produce the chocolate curls.

NUTRITION: Calories: 465 | Carbs: 46.3g | Fat: 28.9g | Protein: 4.4g | Cholesterol: 78mg

---

Herbed Cheesecake

Prep Time: 15 min
Cook Time: 55 min
Servings: 24

- 3 packages (8 ounces each) cream cheese, softened
- 2 cups (16 ounces) sour cream, divided
- 1 can (10-3/4 ounces) condensed cream of celery soup, undiluted
- 3 eggs
- 1/2 cup grated Romano cheese
- 3 garlic cloves, minced
- 1 tablespoon cornstarch
- 2 tablespoons minced fresh basil or 2 teaspoons dried basil
- 1 tablespoon minced fresh thyme or 1 teaspoon dried thyme
- 1/2 teaspoon Italian seasoning
- 1/2 teaspoon coarsely ground pepper
- Assorted crackers

1. Beat soup, a cup of sour cream, and cream cheese in a big bowl until smooth. Beat in pepper, eggs, Italian seasoning, Romano cheese, thyme, garlic, basil, and cornstarch until combined.
2. Transfer to a greased nine-inch springform pan then put the pan on a baking sheet. Bake for 55-60mins in a 350 degrees oven until nearly set in the middle. Cool for 10mins on a wire rack. Slide a knife carefully around the edge of the pan to loosen the cheesecake. Cool for another hour.
3. Chill for at least four hours to overnight; remove the pan sides. Slather the remaining sour cream on top. Serve the cheesecake with crackers. Chill any leftovers.

NUTRITION: Calories: 142 Cal | Cholesterol: 66mg | Protein: 4g | Total Fat: 12g fat | Sodium: 183mg | Fiber: 0 | Carbohydrate: 3g

Desserts and Fruits

Neapolitan Lemon Cookies

Prep Time: 20 min
Cook Time: 20 min
Servings: 24

INGREDIENTS

COOKIE DOUGH
- ½ cup Granulated Sugar
- ¾ of a stick of Butter
- 3 large Eggs
- 1 tablespoon Lemon Extract
- 2 cups All Purpose Flour
- Baking Powder
- 1/8 teaspoon Salt

FROSTING
- 2 ½ cups Confectioners Sugar
- 1 teaspoon Lemon Extract & ¼ cup Water

DIRECTIONS

1. Preheat oven to 325 degrees. Grease a cookie sheet with Crisco or pan spray.
2. In an electric mixer, cream together the ¾ of a stick of Butter, the Sugar, and Lemon Extract until fluffy, about 4 minutes.
3. With mixer on slow speed add eggs 1 and mix until the egg is completed incorporated. Add the second egg and mix until incorporated and do the same with the 3rd egg.
4. Mix salt, flour, and Baking powder together in a smaller bowl. Mix the flour slowly into the egg mixture in three equal parts one at a time.
5. If you have a small scooper (or Tablespoon), scoop some dough onto the cookie pan 1 at a time until all the dough is used up.
6. Bake cookies in oven at 325 degrees until the cookies just barely start getting lightly brown on the edges, about 12-15 minutes. Remove from the oven and let cook on the side.
7. For frosting, combine the Confectioners Sugar, water, and Lemon Extract and mix until smooth. Frost the tops of the cookies. Let the frosting dry a few minutes before serving.

Zabaione

Prep Time: 20 min
Cook Time: 0 min
Servings: 8

- 8 Egg Yolks
- ½ cup Granulated Sugar
- 1 cup Sweet Marsala Wine
- 1 pint fresh Strawberries, washed and quartered
- 9 Ladyfingers (optional)

DIRECTIONS

1. To make this dish you need a double boiler. You can make one by placing a medium pot filled half-way with water, and placing over it a stainless steal mixing bowl that is wider than the pot, so when its place on top of the pot, it won't fall into the pot, but set on top of it.
2. To make the Zabione, have the water in the pot come to the boil, then lower the heat so the water is at a slight simmer. Place the SS Bowl on top of the pot and add the Egg Yolks, Sugar, and Marsala Wine to the bowl.
3. Beat with a Wire Whip until the contents becomes a thick creamy fluffy custard, about 7-8 minutes.
4. Break all the Ladyfingers in half and place 3 pieces in each of 6 Wine Glasses. Equally distribute the Strawberries into the 6 glasses. Fill each glass to the top with Zabaione and serve.

Italian Layer Cake

Prep Time: 15 min
Cook Time: 30 min
Servings: 4

- 16 oz. sponge cake
- 3 1/2 oz. apricot marmalade
- 1 cup Strega liqueur
- 16 oz. whipped cream
- 3 1/2 oz. candied fruit
- 20 oz. cream
- Chocolate bits
- Some cherries

Ingredients for cream:
- 3 egg yolks
- 2 cups milk
- 1 1/2 oz. all-purpose flour
- 1 lemon rind

Cream: Mix the ingredients for cream together. Cook over medium heat, stirring constantly, until ready for cake.

Cake: Cut sponge cake lengthwise in two layers and pour the Strega liqueur over bottom layer with cream, chocolate bits and marmalade. Cover with the remaining cake layer and top with whipped cream, candied fruit and cherries. Serve cold.

Poached Pears

Prep Time: 15 min
Cook Time: 22 min
Servings: 4

- 8 large Bartlett or Anjou Pears
- 6 cups Red Wine
- 1 ½ cups Sugar
- 3 whole Cinnamon Sticks, 10 whole Cloves
- 3 cups Water

1. Peel the Pears, being careful to try and keep the stem on. Place all ingredients in a pot that is large enough to fit all the pears, wine, water, and sugar.
2. Bring liquid to the boil, then lower flame to low and poach the pears for about 18-22 minutes, until you can easily pierce the pears with a fork.
3. Remove the pears from the pot and place in a serving bowl or platter.
4. Strain the Cloves and Cinnamon and discard. Put the pot of poaching liquid back on the stove. Cook over medium heat until the cooking liquid becomes of a syrupy consistency.
5. Serve each person a Poached Pear and drizzle an ample amount of Wine Sauce over each Pear. You can serve as is, with Vanilla Ice Cream or Gelato.

Biscotti

Prep Time: 15 min
Cook Time: 25 min
Servings: 42

INGREDIENTS
- 1/2 cup vegetable oil
- 3 eggs
- 1 cup white sugar
- 1 tablespoon baking powder
- 3 1/4 cups all-purpose flour
- 3 drops anise oil

1. Preheat the oven to 375°F (190°C) (190 degrees C). Line cookie sheets with parchment paper or grease them.
2. Combine the oil, eggs, sugar, and anise flavoring in a medium mixing bowl and whisk until completely combined. To make a heavy dough, combine the flour and baking powder and add to the egg mixture. Divide the dough into two equal parts. Make a rollout of each piece that is as long as your cookie sheet. Place the roll on the prepared cookie sheet and push it down to a thickness of 1/2 inch.

NUTRITION: Calories: 83 Cal | Carbohydrates: 12.3g | Fat: 13g | Protein: 1.4g | Cholesterol: 13mg

Desserts and Fruits

Italian Cheesecake

Prep Time 30 min

Cook Time 2-3 hours and 15 min

Servings 4

INGREDIENTS

- 2 lbs. whole milk Ricotta
- 6 extra large Eggs
- ¾ cup Sugar
- zest of 2 Lemon and 1 Oranges
- 1/8 teaspoon of Salt
- 1 teaspoon Vanilla Extract
- 4 tablespoons flour
- 1-2 cup plain breadcrumbs & 2 tablespoons Sugar
- Butter (to grease pan)

1. Grease a 9" spring-form pan with butter. Mix bread- crumbs and 2 tablespoons of sugar together. Place mixture in buttered pan. Move breadcrumb mixture around to coat pan with mixture.
2. Beat eggs with ¾ cup of sugar. Add vanilla, and Lemon & Orange Zest if using. Add flour and continue beating ingredients together. Little by little, add the Ricotta to bowl and mix until all the ricotta is incorporated and smooth.
3. Heat oven to 375 degrees.
4. Place the spring-form pan inside a large pan. Pour all of the Ricotta (Cheesecake) mixture inside the spring-form pan. Pour warm water into the larger pan that is holding the spring-form pan with the ricotta mixture. Pour water half way up the sides of the spring-form pan. This is a water-bath.
5. Bake for 15 minute at 375 degrees. Turn oven down to 325 degree and bake cheesecake for 50 to 60 minutes more, until when you put a toothpick into the center of the cake, it comes out clean.
6. Cool cheesecake for 1 hour outside at room temperature. Place cheesecake in refrigerator and cook for 2 to 3 hours before serving.

Italian Rice Pudding

Prep Time 20 min

Cook Time 25 min

Servings 8

INGREDIENTS

- 2 cups Arborio Rice
- 2 ½ cups of Milk
- ½ cup Sugar, 3 large Eggs, beaten
- 1 tablespoon melted Butter
- 1/8 teaspoon Salt, Zest of 1 Orange
- ¼ cup Raisons
- ¼ teaspoon each of Cinnamon and Nutmeg

DIRECTIONS

1. Place 4 quarts of water in a 6 quart pot and bring to the boil. Add the rice and boil for 14 minutes. Remove from heat and strain the rice in a wire-strainer. Run cold water over and into the rice for 5 minutes. Shake off excess water and let the rice sit and cool for 12 minutes.
2. Place the beaten Eggs, Milk, Salt, melted Butter, Raisons, and Orange Zest in a large bowl and mix. Add the rice and mix.
3. Turn oven on to 350 degrees. Place the rice into a 9" X 13" Pyrex baking pan and bake in the oven at 350 degrees for 20 minutes. Remove from the oven and let cool on the counter. Sprinkle Cinnamon and Nutmeg over the top of the pudding and put into the refrigerator at least 3 hours before serving.

NUTRITION: Calories: 11Cal | Carbohydrates: 2.6g | Fat: 0.1g | Protein: 0.6g | Cholesterol: 0mg

Italian Almond Pie

Prep Time: 15 min
Cook Time: 50 min
Servings: 8

INGREDIENTS

- 1 teaspoon cardamom
- ½ teaspoon ground clove
- 1 teaspoon ground anise
- 1 teaspoon vanilla extract
- 1 egg, beaten
- 1-pound pie crust
- 4 tablespoon almond paste
- 8 oz pears
- ¼ cup brown sugar
- 1 teaspoon cinnamon
- 4 tablespoon lemon juice
- 1 tablespoon butter
- ½ cup almond flakes

DIRECTIONS

1. Roll the pie crust carefully.
2. Then spread the form with the butter and put the rolled pie crust there.
3. After this, slice the pears and sprinkle them with the lemon juice to avoid the dark spots on the fruits.
4. Put the fruits in the pie form.
5. Combine the brown sugar, cinnamon, cardamom, ground clove, and ground anise in the shallow bowl. Stir it gently with the fork.
6. After this, sprinkle the spice mixture over the sliced pears.
7. Add the vanilla extract.
8. Whisk the egg and brush the surface of the pie.
9. Then make the layer of the almond flakes over the pie.
10. Preheat the oven to 365 F.
11. Put the pear pie in the oven and bake it for 50 minutes.
12. Then remove the pie from the oven and let it cool briefly.
13. Discard the pie from the form.

Nutrition: Calories 357 Cal | Fat 20.1g | Fiber 2g | Carbohydrates 39g | Protein 5g

---

Italian cream Hot Chocolate

Prep Time: 5 min
Cook Time: 8 min
Servings: 4

INGREDIENTS

- 1 teaspoon vanilla sugar
- 1 cup cream
- 4 tablespoon milk
- 10 oz dark chocolate
- 1 tablespoon brown sugar
- 1 teaspoon potato starch

DIRECTIONS

1. Melt the chocolate in the water bath.
2. When the dark chocolate is liquid – add brown sugar and vanilla sugar.
3. Whisk the mixture until sugar is dissolved.
4. After this, combine milk with the potato starch and whisk it until homogenous.
5. Then add cream to the melted dark chocolate mixture and stir it gently.
6. When you get homogenous mass – pour the potato starch liquid slowly into the mixture.
7. Whisk it carefully.
8. Chill the cooked hot chocolate for 5 minutes.

Nutrition: Calories 580 | Fat 33.4 | Fiber 7 | Carbos 61.52 | Protein 9

Desserts and Fruits

Cream Lemon Pie vanilla

Prep Time 15 min   **Cook Time** 40 min   **Servings** 10

INGREDIENTS

- 1 teaspoon vanilla extract
- 1 teaspoon salt
- 1 teaspoon cinnamon
- 1 tablespoon lemon zest
- 1 teaspoon butter
- 1 cup cream
- 3 cup flour
- 5 eggs
- 1 cup sugar
- ½ tablespoon baking soda

1. Crack the eggs into the bowl and whisk them well.
2. Add sugar and whisk the liquid until you get lemon color.
3. After this, add cream and mix the mixture with the help of the hand mixer.
4. Then add flour, salt, vanilla extract, cinnamon, lemon zest, and baking soda.
5. Knead the smooth and liquid dough.
6. Preheat the oven to 365 F.
7. Spread the cake form with the butter inside.
8. Then pour the dough into the form and place in the oven.
9. Bake the cream lemon pie for 40 minutes. Check if it is done with the help of the toothpick.
10. Remove the cooked pie from the oven and chill it very well.

Nutrition: Calories 293 Cal | Fat 10.2g | Fiber 1g | Carbs 40.35g | Protein 9g

---

Chocolate Salami

Prep Time 1 hour and 20 min   **Cook Time** 7 min   **Servings** 8

INGREDIENTS

- 4 tablespoon caster sugar
- 8 oz biscuits
- ¼ cup hazelnuts
- ½ cup peanuts
- 12 oz dark chocolate
- 1 teaspoon amaretto
- 1 cup butter
- ¼ cup sugar
- 3 tablespoon cocoa powder
- 4 egg

DIRECTIONS

1. Melt the dark chocolate and combine it with amaretto.
2. Stir the mixture and chill it.
3. Meanwhile, beat the eggs in the mixer bowl and add butter.
4. Mix the mass up until you get a fluffy texture.
5. Then add sugar and continue to mix it for 1 minute more.
6. Combine the mixed butter mass with the chilled dark chocolate and stir it with the help of the spoon.
7. After this, crush the hazelnuts and peanuts.
8. Add the nuts to the chocolate mixture. Knead it.
9. Then transfer the chocolate mass on the plastic wrap and roll it up to make the shape of the sausage.
10. Put the chocolate sausage in the freezer and leave it there for 1 hour.
11. After this, discard the chocolate sausage from the freezer and make it dry with the help of the paper towel.
12. Sprinkle the chocolate sausage with the caster sugar and slice it.
13. Serve the dessert!

NUTRITION: Calories 746 Cal | Fat 52.7g | Fiber 6g | Carbohydrates 56.7g | Protein 15g |

Almond Cake

Prep Time: 10 min
Cook Time: 40 min
Servings: 10

INGREDIENTS

- Zest from 1 orange, grated
- 1 and ¼ cups sugar
- 6 eggs, whites and yolks separated
- ½ pound almonds, blanched and ground
- Zest from 1 lemon, grated
- 4 drops almond extract
- Confectioner's sugar

DIRECTIONS

1. Beat egg yolks with your mixer very well.
2. Add sugar, almond extract, orange and lemon zest and almonds and stir well.
3. Beat egg whites in another bowl with your mixer.
4. Add egg yolks mix and stir everything.
5. Pour this into a greased baking dish, introduce in the oven at 350 degrees F and bake for 40 minutes.
6. Take cake out of the oven, leave it to cool down, slice, dust confectioners' sugar on top and serve.

NUTRITION: Calories 200 Cal | Fat 0 | Fiber 0 | Carbos 23g | Protein 6g

---

Star Anise Biscotti

Prep Time: 15 min
Cook Time: 50 min
Servings: 20

INGREDIENTS

- ¾ cup (180 ml) granulated sugar
- 1/3 cup (80 ml) room temperature almond milk
- 2 tablespoons (30 ml) melted vegan butter
- 1 teaspoon (5 ml) anisette liqueur
- 2 ¼ cups (555 ml) all-purpose flour
- 1 teaspoon (5 ml) baking powder
- 2 teaspoons (10 ml) anise seed
- 1/3 cup (80 ml) walnuts, chopped

DIRECTIONS

1. Program your oven 350° F (175° C), then line a cookie sheet with parchment paper.
2. Whisk the granulated sugar, almond milk, melted butter, and anisette liqueur in a large bowl.
3. Place a sieve over a separate bowl, add the all-purpose flour, baking powder, and salt and sift into the bowl.
4. Next, add the flour baking powder mixture to the sugar almond mixture and mix until a shaggy dough forms.
5. Add the anise seeds and walnuts to the dough and mix until they are evenly incorporated, then shape into a dough ball.
6. Divide the biscotti into two even portions and shape each portion into a log that is 2 inches (5 cm) in length.
7. Transfer the biscotti to the prepared cookie sheet, spaced a few inches/cm apart, and carefully flatten them slightly.
8. Bake the biscotti for 32-35 minutes until firm and slightly browned.
9. Remove the biscotti from the oven and allow to cool for 12-15 minutes.
10. Decrease the oven's temperature to 275° F (135° C), and carefully cut the logs into ½ inch (1.5 cm) wide diagonal slices using a serrated-edged knife.
11. Arrange the star anise biscotti slices cut side down on the cookie sheet and bake for an additional 8 minutes.
12. Place the star anise biscotti onto a wire rack to cool completely.
13. Serve and enjoy!

Desserts and Fruits

Orange And Hazelnut Cake

Prep Time 10 min | **Cook Time** 40 min | **Servings** 10

INGREDIENTS

For the syrup:
- 2 and ½ tablespoons orange juice
- 1 and ¼ cups sugar
- 2/3 cup water
- 2 and ½ tablespoons orange water
- Zest from 1 orange, grated

For the cake:
- 2 and ¼ cups hazelnut flour
- 5 eggs, whites and yolks separated
- 1 cup sugar
- 2 tablespoons confectioners' sugar for serving
- 1 and 1/3 cups Greek yogurt for serving
- Pulp from 4 passion fruits

DIRECTIONS

1. Put the water in a pot and bring to a boil over medium high heat.
2. Add orange juice and 1 and ¼ cups sugar, stir and boil for 10 minutes.
3. Take off heat, add orange zest and orange water, stir and leave aside.
4. In a bowl, beat egg yolks with 1 cup sugar and hazelnut flour using your mixer.
5. In another bowl, beat egg whites using your mixer as well.
6. Combine the 2 mixtures and stir well.
7. Pour this batter into a greased and lined baking form, introduce in the oven at 350 degrees F and bake for 30 minutes.
8. Take cake out of the oven, leave it to cool down a bit, slice and serve with the orange sauce you've made, with yogurt, confectioners' sugar dusted on top and passion fruit pulp on the side.

NUTRITION: Calories 234 Cal | Fat 1g | Fiber 2g | Carbos 4g | Protein 7g

---

Savory Tomato Pie

Prep Time 25 min | **Cook Time** 45 min | **Servings** 8

INGREDIENTS

- 5 green onions, sliced
- 3/4 cup chopped sweet onion
- 2 tablespoons butter
- 2 pounds tomatoes, peeled, seeded and chopped
- 1 unbaked pastry shell (9 inches)
- 3 eggs
- 1 cup half-and-half cream
- 1-1/2 teaspoons salt
- 1 tablespoon minced fresh basil or 1 teaspoon dried basil
- 1/2 teaspoon white pepper

DIRECTIONS

1. Sauté onions in a big pan with butter until tender; put in tomatoes. On low heat, cook and stir until soft. Take off heat then cool.
2. Place a double-thick heavy-duty foil on unbaked pastry shell. Bake for 5mins in a 450 degrees oven. Discard the foil then bake for another 5mins. Lower heat to 350 degrees.
3. Beat pepper, eggs, basil, salt, and cream in a bowl until smooth; combine with the tomato mixture. Pour the mixture in the pastry shell then bake for 45-50mins until an inserted knife in the middle comes out without residue. Let it sit for 5mins then slice.

NUTRITION: Calories: 246 | Total Fat: 15g | Sodium: 622mg | Fiber: 2g | Total Carbohydrate: 22g | Cholesterol: 107mg | Protein: 6g

Italian Chocolate Cake

Prep Time 50 min

Cook Time 25 min

Servings 6

INGREDIENTS

For the chocolate cake
- 1 ½ cups (360 ml) all-purpose flour
- 1 cup (235 ml) granulated sugar
- ½ cup (120 ml) dark chocolate cocoa powder
- 1 teaspoon (5 ml) baking soda
- ¼ teaspoon (1.25 ml) salt
- 1/3 cup (80 ml) olive oil
- 1 tablespoon (15 ml) balsamic vinegar
- 1 tablespoon (15 ml) pure vanilla bean paste
- 1 cup (235 ml) almond milk
- 4 tablespoons (60 ml) espresso, cooled

For the chocolate icing:
- ¾ cup (180 ml) dark chocolate, chopped
- ½ cup (113 g/120 ml) vegan butter
- 2 tablespoons (30 ml) olive oil
- 1 tablespoon (15 ml) vanilla bean paste

DIRECTIONS

1. Position the oven's rack in the center of the oven, and program your oven to 350° F (175° C).
2. Coat a 9 inch (23 cm) circular cake pan with nonstick cooking spray or butter and flour, then line with parchment paper.
3. Sift the all-purpose flour, cocoa, baking soda, and salt into a large mixing bowl.
4. Whisk the olive oil, balsamic vinegar, vanilla bean paste, almond milk, and coffee in a separate bowl.
5. Add the olive oil mixture to the flour cocoa mixture and mix just until combined.
6. Pour the chocolate cake batter into the prepared pan and bake for 40 minutes until a skewer comes out clean.
7. Allow the chocolate cake to cool in the pan for 10 minutes, then invert onto a wire rack.
8. Place about an inch (2.5 cm) of water into a saucepot and allow to come to a simmer over medium-high heat.
9. Add the dark chocolate and butter to a heat-safe bowl, place over the pot of simmering water, and stir the chocolate and butter constantly until melted.
10. Remove the chocolate-butter mixture from the pot and whisk in the olive oil and vanilla bean paste.
11. Allow the frosting to cool completely until the icing is thick enough to frost the cake.
12. Frost the chocolate cake with the chocolate icing and top with more chopped dark chocolate if desired.
13. Serve and enjoy.

Desserts and Fruits

21 Days Meal Plan

21 Days	Breakfast	Main Dish	Side Dish	Dessert
Day 1	Italian Mini Frittatas	Swordfish in Red Sauce	Rice Cake	Sicilian Chocolate Cake
Day 2	Breakfast Risotto	White Bean Crostini	Hot Rice Salad	Zabaoine
Day 3	Italian Strata	Zucchini Tomato Soup	Creamy Rice with Porcini	Savory Biscuits
Day 4	Italian Mini Frittatas	Turkey Cutlets	Italian Rice Pie	Poached Pears
Day 5	Ricotta Pancakes	Beefy Italian Ramen Skillet	Rice Cake	Artichoke Pizza
Day 6	Italian Brunch Torte	Italian Potato Soup	Cherry Tomato Salad	Herb Bread
Day 7	Simple Italian Omelet	Zucchini Crepes	Italian Jasmine Rice	Watermelon Granita
Day 8	Italian Strata	Stewed Eggplants and Tomatoes	Eggplant Pasta	Herbed Cheesecake
Day 9	Ricotta Pancakes	Easy Beef Braciole	Rice with olives	Almond Italian Cookies
Day 10	Egg and Tomato Scramble	Pan Fried Asparagus	Classic Paella Simple	Zabaione
Day 11	Breakfast Couscous	Roast Sicilian Rabbit	Sicilian Salad	Biscotti
Day 12	Meatball sandwich	Rabbit Stew	Italian Rice Pie	Apple Strudel
Day 13	Caramelized Mushroom and Onion Frittata	Italian Lamb	Milanese style Risotto	Star Anise Biscotti
Day 14	Italian Strata	Italian Pork Tenderloin	Cherry Tomato Salad	Savory Tomato Pie
Day 15	Italian Aromatic Breakfast Bombs	Lemon Chicken Piccata	Pepperoni pasta	Italian Layer Cake
Day 16	Italian Breakfast Casserole	Italian-Style Baked Zucchini	Creamy Rice with Porcini	Italian Almond Pie
Day 17	Italian Strata	Chicken Fettuccini Alfredo	Sweet Sour Pasta Salad	Apple Strudel
Day 18	Ricotta Pancakes	Italian Halibut Chowder	Crispy Cauliflower	Fresh Orange Gelato
Day 19	Italian Brunch Torte	Zucchini and Corn stuffed Chicken	Tofu Spinach Lasagna	Zabaione
Day 20	Simple Italian omelet	Pan Chicken with Tomato	Italian Jasmine Rice	Almond Cake
Day 21	Meatball Sandwich	Balsamic Vinegar Steak	Seashell Salad	Savory Biscuits

CONCLUSION

Italian food is a true commodity event, and nutrition is a secondary consideration. A traditional Italian meal begins with a large plate of antipasti, mostly vegetables (such as pepperoncini, artichoke hearts, and mushrooms) and a choice of grilled meat. Then it goes on to a tiny pasta dish accompanied by a lighter protein, maybe a leg of lamb, cooked easily but delightfully. It gets easier as the meal continues. Italian dinners tend to have a crescendo in turn.

The core of most Italian cuisine is olive oil; then, the veggies move in. Onion and garlic are the usual go-to, but the plate's highlights are also intense green veggies. In Italian cuisine, balsamic vinegar still demands a prime location, and you will be hard pushed to find a chef within easy reach without a slice of Grana Padano. The Italians are huge fans of preserving to turn bacon into salami and sausage, grapes into liquor, and onions into pickled vegetables. When you are trying to make the tastiness last, they are true believers in spending the effort.

With flavorful vegetables such as tomatoes, sweet potato, eggplant, and good oil sources, such as olives or canola oil, many new Italian appetizers are made. You will enjoy a vegetable soup or antipasto salad, a small pasta section, and a fatty protein and vegetable entree if you keep the serving sizes small. It would certainly not come as a shock that you won't do much with your waistline with the starchy, fluffy pasta you find on most Italian lists. The nutrition of Italian food would also depend on where you want to dine. Owing to the addition of spaghetti, Italian cuisine appears to be rich in carbs, although some low-carbohydrate choices may exist. Based on ingredients, precise nutritional standards differ.

For all its followers, Italian food has always succeeded in creating a fine dining experience. You will also need to have the right equipment in your hand if you love making delicious Italian meals.

Printed in Great Britain
by Amazon